Julie Stafford's
Sweets

VIKING

Viking
Penguin Books Australia Ltd
487 Maroondah Highway, PO Box 257
Ringwood, Victoria 3134, Australia
Penguin Books Ltd
Harmondsworth, Middlesex, England
Viking Penguin, A Division of Penguin Books USA Inc.
375 Hudson Street, New York, New York 10014, USA
Penguin Books Canada Limited
10 Alcorn Avenue, Toronto, Ontario, Canada M4V 3B2
Penguin Books (N.Z.) Ltd
Cnr Rosedale and Airborne Roads, Albany, Auckland, New Zealand

First published by Penguin Books Australia Ltd 1997

10 9 8 7 6 5 4 3 2 1

Copyright © Julie Stafford, 1997

Design by Limor Gilboa, Penguin Design Studio
Photography by John Hay
Food preparation and styling by Fiona Hammond
Illustrations by Michelle Ryan
Typeset in 11.5/20pt Bembo by Post Typesetters, Queensland
Printed in Australia by Australian Print Group, Maryborough, Victoria

National Library of Australia
Cataloguing-in-Publication data

Stafford, Julie.
    Julie Stafford's sweets.

    Includes index.
    ISBN 0 670 86771 3.

    1. Desserts. 2. Sugar-free confectionery. 3. Sugar-free diet – Recipes.
    4. Low-fat diet – Recipes. I. Title. II. Title: Sweets.

641.86

FRONT COVER PHOTOGRAPH
Baked Berry Cheesecake with Raspberry Sauce
(see page 4).

CONTENTS

Introduction   *iv*

Cakes, Slices & Tortes   1

Fruit, Glorious Fruit   21

Ice-creams & Sorbets   37

Mousses, Jellies & Fruit Swirls   51

Pies & Puddings   61

Tarts, Flans & Galettes   77

Sauces & Custards   97

Pastry & Other Basic Recipes   105

About the Ingredients   *111*

Index   *118*

INTRODUCTION

I grew up in a home where a meal was not complete without a sweet offering of some sort being served. It could have been a cake or slice, trifle, pavlova, cream-filled pastry and sponge, apple pie, hot jam pudding, rich fruit pudding or golden syrup dumplings to ward off the winter chills, cheesecake, or, a favourite, gingernut lemon pie. I drooled at the look of these sometimes simple and sometimes extravagant sweet treats. I loved the warm feelings they'd suggest; you knew you were going to be just a little spoilt or loved, and the sweet, creamy, sticky, spicy, tart, tangy, tasty experiences were nearly always to die for. When I look closely at the ingredients of some of those childhood dishes I am amazed that my arteries are not totally clogged, and I have not actually died of dessert-related disease!

Although the primary purpose of food is to nourish, there is something quite special about the wonderful memories that a sweet offering evokes. Try as hard as I might, the same warm memories do not come flooding back when I think of a pot of soup, a casserole, a tossed salad or even a sandwich.

Just mention the word 'lamington' and I can immediately recall a busy kitchen full of wonderful aromas, a bench covered with chequered tea towels, and bright yellow sponge squares lined up precisely like soldiers ready for some military manoeuvre, a big bowl of chocolate sauce, forks leaning against the side, an even bigger bowl of coconut and the question on everyone's lips, 'How long before they are ready to eat, Mum?'.

My mother was a fabulous cook, especially of desserts, cakes and all sorts of sweet treats. Her pavlovas were crunchy on the outside, chewy on the inside, and topped with lots of cream, strawberries, passionfruit and pineapple. Every mouth-watering spoonful was a memory in itself.

Mum would always double the mixture and we would wait patiently (and sometimes not so) for the invitation to go back for seconds!

The making of melt-in-your-mouth shortbread, the smell of spicy mince pies, Christmas cake and Christmas pudding (with threepences of course) meant that Christmas was coming.

Trifle reminds me of long Sunday roast lunches with all the family, where you really had to stretch your appetite and often loosen your belt to fit any more in. But you wouldn't think of leaving the table without just a little dessert!

Chocolate sponges filled with cream and strawberries meant that it was someone's birthday and a time to be home to help celebrate it. The same sponge came filled with lashings of cream and was topped with dozens of small chocolate eggs for Easter. And it didn't matter how hard you tried – you could never cut the cake in such a way so that each portion had the same number of eggs.

Finding hedgehogs or some jam rolypoly in the school lunch box would brighten up even the worst day at school.

Steamed jam and fruit puddings conjure up a vision of Mum standing in front of the old wood stove sorting through the selection of wood blocks, deciding which pieces of wood would keep the pressure cooker steaming for just the right length of time to turn out a moist, delicious pudding. She did it every time, too.

My Gran taught me at a very early age that the best way to remember how to differentiate between the words desert and dessert on a spelling test was to remember the double 'ss' in dessert represented double helpings . . . a chance to go back a second time and indulge oneself. I confess I have been known to do this once or twice . . . in the past, naturally.

Two of my very favourite food experiences have been to wander the dessert section of Harrod's Food Hall in London and Balducci's delicatessen in New York. These places leave you in total awe of all the dessert possibilities that can be created using simple ingredients like flour, eggs, butter, sugar, cream and, nearly always, chocolate!

Although I could really let my hair down in the kitchen using these typical dessert and sweet treat ingredients, *Sweets* is intended to bring you sweet recipe ideas loaded with taste but without the saturated fat and sugar that most often take desserts and sweet treats off the menu for those on a low-fat diet.

In this book you'll find traditional favourites with a healthy twist and lots of new ideas for cakes, slices, puddings, pies, tarts, tortes, strudels, fruit desserts, sauces and even ice-creams.

A sweet offering can still be the perfect balance to a main meal. Serve the very low-fat recipes, especially the fruit recipe ideas, after a heavy main meal. The more substantial sweet recipes like puddings, pies and tortes are delightful after a light main meal or enjoy them for a Sunday brunch or a lazy Sunday supper.

CAKES, SLICES & TORTES

The cake has changed. No longer are we satisfied with a light, cream-filled sponge or plain butter cake topped with lemon icing, or a fruit loaf buttered hot from the oven. Just walk into any coffee or cake shop and you'll find poppyseed cake topped with sticky orange syrup; chunky pineapple, date and banana cake topped with caramelised coconut; or rich and mud-like chocolate cake.

Today the art of cake-making defies all the basic rules and the cakes here are no exception. You'll find most of them have a fruit or even vegetable content to give them a lovely, moist, sweet taste. The saturated fat ingredients like butter, cream and egg yolks normally found in cake recipes have either been removed, replaced with another more suitable low-fat ingredient, or the amount used has been reduced to make these recipes healthier. Yes, you can have your cake and eat it!

APPLE & HAZELNUT CUSTARD CAKE

A moist cake that combines the flavours of hazelnuts, mixed spice and apples.

1 cup unbleached self-raising flour

1 cup unbleached wholemeal self-
   raising flour

1 teaspoon mixed spice

¾ cup finely ground hazelnuts

450 g chopped cooked Granny Smith
   apples or unsweetened canned
   pie apples

½ cup apple juice concentrate

¼ cup grapeseed oil

¾ cup low-fat milk or soymilk

2 whole eggs or 3 egg whites

1 tablespoon vanilla essence

2 cups Basic Custard (see page 99)

- Preheat the oven to 180°C. Line a round 25 cm cake tin with baking paper.

- Sift the flours and mixed spice into a bowl. Fold in the hazelnuts and add the apple.

- In another bowl, combine the apple juice concentrate, grapeseed oil, milk, eggs and vanilla essence. Beat well and fold into the flour and apple mixture.

- Spoon into the prepared tin and bake for 50 minutes.

- Allow the cake to cool slightly before turning out onto a cooling rack. When cake is cool, cut in half and fill with the cooled custard.

APRICOT CRUMBLE SLICE

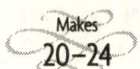

Makes
20–24

This crumble can be served as a warm dessert with Citrus Custard (see page 101) or cold as an afternoon tea slice.

1 quantity Sweet Pastry (see page 107)
or ½ quantity Wholemeal Almond
Pastry (see page 108)

FILLING
250 g dried apricots
1 cup water
1 teaspoon finely grated orange zest

TOPPING
2 egg whites
125 g almonds, finely ground
1 teaspoon vanilla essence
2 tablespoons apple juice concentrate
2 tablespoons shredded coconut

- Firmly press the pastry into a lined 20 cm × 30 cm slice tin and set aside.

- To make the Filling, place the apricots, water and orange zest in a saucepan and gently poach until the apricots are soft, about 15–20 minutes.

- Purée the mixture and allow to cool slightly before spreading over the pastry base.

- Preheat the oven to 180°C.

- To make the Topping, beat the egg whites until stiff. Fold in all the other ingredients in the order they are listed and spoon over the apricots.

- Cook for 20–25 minutes or until the top is firm and lightly brown. Cool the pie in the tin before slicing.

BAKED BERRY CHEESECAKE WITH RASPBERRY SAUCE

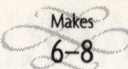
Makes
6–8

400 g low-fat cottage cheese

500 g low-fat ricotta

2 tablespoons unbleached plain flour

¼ cup apple juice concentrate

1 teaspoon cinnamon

2 eggs

2 egg whites

2 cups mixed berries (blackberries, blueberries, raspberries)

1 quantity Raspberry Sauce (see page 104)

extra fresh berries for decorating

- Preheat the oven to 170°C. Line the base and sides of a round 20 cm cheesecake tin with removable sides with baking paper.

- Purée the first 7 ingredients until smooth and creamy. Fold in the berries.

- Pour the mixture into the prepared tin and bake for 30–40 minutes or until the cheesecake is firm in the centre (test with a skewer, which should come out clean). Remove from the oven and allow to cool in the tin.

- Turn out the cheesecake onto a serving platter and chill before serving. Serve with raspberry sauce and extra fresh berries.

BANANA, BOURBON & ORANGE CAKE

Serves
10–12

The smell of bourbon, cinnamon and orange that wafts from the oven when the cake is baking is reason alone to make it. It is moist in the middle, slightly crispy on the outside and can be served hot with Orange Citrus Sauce (see page 103) or yoghurt, garnished with long strips of fresh orange zest.

1 cup unbleached wholemeal self-
   raising flour

1 cup unbleached self-raising flour

1/2 teaspoon bicarbonate of soda

1 teaspoon cinnamon

3 bananas, peeled and diced

1 orange, peeled and chopped

2 tablespoons bourbon

1/2 cup apple juice concentrate

1/2 cup grapeseed oil

3/4 cup freshly squeezed orange juice

2 eggs or 3 egg whites

- Preheat the oven to 180°C. Line a rectangular loaf tin with baking paper.

- Sift the dry ingredients into a mixing bowl and add the bananas, orange and bourbon.

- Combine the apple juice concentrate, grapeseed oil and orange juice. Fold into the flour and fruit mixture.

- Beat the whole eggs or egg whites until they are light and fluffy and fold through the mixture.

- Spoon into the prepared tin and bake for approximately 45 minutes.

- Turn out onto a cooling rack and cover with a tea towel.

BANANA & RHUBARB CAKE

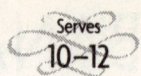

Serves
10–12

This is an ideal recipe for times when rhubarb and bananas are plentiful. This cake is loaded with energy and taste, and can be served warm or cold with Citrus Custard (see page 101) or ice-cream.

1½ cups unbleached white self-raising flour	½ cup grapeseed oil
1 cup wholemeal plain flour	½ cup apple juice concentrate
1 teaspoon cinnamon	¾ cup low-fat soymilk or skim milk
300 g rhubarb, finely chopped	2 whole eggs or 3 egg whites
3 bananas, peeled and mashed	50 g almonds

- Preheat the oven to 180°C. Line a round 25 cm cake tin with baking paper.

- Sift the flours and cinnamon into a bowl and add the rhubarb and banana.

- In another bowl, combine the grapeseed oil, apple juice concentrate, milk and eggs. Beat well and fold into the banana mixture.

- Spoon into the prepared tin and top with almonds. Bake for 45 minutes.

- Allow the cake to cool slightly before turning out onto a cooling rack.

BERRY STREUSEL CAKE

Serves
10–12

This is a deliciously moist cake with a spicy, nutty topping. The raspberries and blueberries work well together, but you can use other berry combinations. Do not use canned berries. Serve the cake warm or cold; it is delicious as a dessert with a little whipped ricotta, citrus custard, yoghurt or ice-cream.

1½ cups unbleached self-raising flour

½ cup unbleached plain flour

300 g raspberries, fresh or frozen

300 g blueberries, fresh or frozen

½ cup grapeseed oil

½ cup apple juice concentrate

¾ cup low-fat milk or soymilk

2 whole eggs or 3 egg whites

STREUSEL TOPPING

2 tablespoons shredded coconut

2 tablespoons roughly chopped
  pecans

1 teaspoon cinnamon

1 teaspoon mixed spice

- Preheat the oven to 180°C. Line a square cake tin with baking paper.
- Sift the flours into a bowl and add the berries.
- In another bowl, combine the grapeseed oil, apple juice concentrate, milk and eggs. Beat well and fold into the flour and berries.
- To make the Streusel Topping, combine all the ingredients and mix well.
- Spoon the cake mixture into the prepared tin and top with streusel. Bake for 55 minutes.
- Allow the cake to cool slightly in the tin before turning out onto a cooling rack.

CAROB & DATE MUD CAKE

Serves
12–16

This is possibly my favourite recipe after the Berry Pudding (see page 65). You need only the tiniest sliver to enjoy a sweet experience, and it can be served warm or cold. I like it best with a light dusting of icing sugar and warm raspberry sauce. Keep any leftovers in the refrigerator.

400 g dates, halved

1½ cups boiling water

1 teaspoon bicarbonate of soda

½ cup grapeseed oil

½ cup apple juice concentrate

1 tablespoon vanilla essence

2 cups unbleached plain flour

1 cup carob powder

2 teaspoons mixed spice

1 cup low-fat milk

- Preheat the oven to 170°C. Line a round 20 cm cake tin with baking paper.

- Combine the dates, boiling water and bicarbonate of soda, stir and stand until the mixture has cooled.

- Stir in the grapeseed oil, apple juice concentrate and vanilla essence.

- Sift together the flour, carob powder and mixed spice, and fold into the date mixture. Add the milk and stir to incorporate.

- Spoon into the prepared tin and bake for 55 minutes.

- Allow the cake to cool slightly in the tin before turning out onto a cooling rack.

CAROB HEDGEHOG BALLS

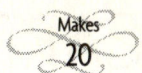

Makes
20

These highly nutritious power-packed balls of energy taste fabulous. For special occasions macerate the fruit in your favourite liqueur or brandy. They are delicious served with a selection of fresh fruits after the main meal. Wrap them in cellophane and hang on the Christmas tree.

The mixture is best made in a food processor. If you have a small-capacity food processor, divide the quantities in half, make two lots of the mixture and combine them by hand.

1 cup dates	*2 cups rolled oats*
1 cup raisins	*2 tablespoons carob powder*
1 cup whole almonds	*2 teaspoons vanilla essence*
1 cup shredded coconut	*3 tablespoons apple juice concentrate*

- Place the dates, raisins, almonds, coconut, rolled oats and carob powder in a food processor and process until the mixture resembles breadcrumbs.

- Add the vanilla essence and apple juice concentrate and continue to process until the mixture begins to stick together.

- Roll into balls the size of 50-cent pieces and keep in the refrigerator.

- The balls can be rolled in extra carob powder or shredded coconut if desired.

CARROT CAKE WITH LEMON CHEESE ICING

Serves
10–12

2 cups finely grated carrot

1 cup sultanas or finely chopped dates
 or finely chopped raisins

1½ teaspoons cinnamon

½ cup freshly squeezed orange juice

½ cup apple juice concentrate

⅓ cup grapeseed oil

1 cup unbleached wholemeal flour

1 cup unbleached plain flour

3 teaspoons baking powder

2 whole eggs or 3 egg whites

shredded coconut or lemon zest
 (garnish)

LEMON CHEESE ICING

1 cup cold Lemon Sauce (see page 101)

100 g low-fat ricotta

- Preheat the oven to 170°C. Line a square or round cake tin with baking paper.

- Place the carrot, sultanas, cinnamon, orange juice and apple juice concentrate in a saucepan and slowly bring to the boil. Cover and gently simmer for a few minutes or until the sultanas, dates or raisins are soft. Remove from the heat and allow the mixture to cool.

- Add the grapeseed oil.

- Sift the flours and baking powder together and fold into the carrot mixture.

- Beat the eggs or egg whites lightly and fold into the mixture.

- Spoon into the prepared tin and bake for 50 minutes.

- Allow the cake to cool slightly in the tin before turning out onto a cooling rack.

- To make the Lemon Cheese Icing, blend all the ingredients until smooth. Refrigerate until the mixture is quite firm.

- Spread the lemon cheese icing over the cooled cake and sprinkle the top with shredded coconut or thin strips of lemon zest.

CHEWY BANANA & NUT SLICE

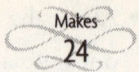

Makes
24

This chewy sweet treat reminds me a little of nougat. It can be eaten as is or sliced thinly and served with fruit after dinner.

200 g dried bananas

100 g dried apples

100 g whole almonds

100 g hazelnuts

125 g rolled oats

30 g shredded coconut

3 tablespoons apple juice concentrate

a squeeze of lemon juice

a little extra shredded coconut

- Process the banana, apple, almonds, hazelnuts, rolled oats and coconut in a food processor until the mixture resembles breadcrumbs.

- Add the apple juice concentrate and lemon juice and continue processing until the mixture begins to stick together.

- Press the mixture into a shallow slice tray lined with non-stick paper and roll out with a straight-sided glass. Press the extra coconut on top of the slice.

- Refrigerate and cut into portions when firm.

CHRISTMAS CAKE

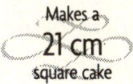

Makes a
21 cm
square cake

*Traditional Christmas fruit-cake recipes tend to be loaded with but-
ter, sugar and whole eggs. Needless to say, a very small slice goes a long
way. This recipe produces a moist, fruity and spicy cake but has no
added fat or refined sugar, and uses only egg whites — ideal for those
who love a big wedge of Christmas cake! It is best made the day
before you are going to eat it. Any leftovers can be kept in the refrigerator to maintain its freshness and moistness.*

125 g dried apricots, chopped

125 g raisins, chopped

125 g mixed dried peel

125 g currants, chopped

125 g stoned prunes or dried figs,
  chopped

225 g stoned dates, chopped

2 tablespoons brandy

1 cup freshly squeezed orange juice

500 g peeled pumpkin, cooked
  and mashed

1/2 cup apple juice concentrate

3 cups unbleached white self-raising
  flour

1 cup unbleached plain wholemeal
  flour

1 teaspoon ground cinnamon

1 teaspoon mixed spice

1/2 teaspoon ground nutmeg

6 egg whites

2 teaspoons vanilla essence

GLAZE

1 cup glacé fruit and nuts

1 cup Cake and Flan Glaze (see
  page 109)

- Soak the fruits in brandy and orange juice. Cover and
  leave to stand overnight.

- Preheat the oven to 160°C. Line the base and sides of a
  deep 21 cm square cake tin with a double layer of
  baking paper. >

- Add the pumpkin and apple juice concentrate to the
  fruit mixture and mix well.

- Sift the flours and spices together and fold into the fruit
  mixture in three lots.

- Beat the egg whites until stiff. Gently fold through the
  fruit mixture and add the vanilla essence. Stir to
  incorporate.

- Spoon into the prepared tin and bake cake for
  2½–3 hours or until a wooden skewer inserted into the
  centre of the cake comes out clean.

- Cool in the tin before topping with the glazed fruit
  and nuts.

- To make the Glaze, add the glacé fruit and nuts to the
  cake and flan glaze and cook as per page 109. With a pair
  of tongs, position the fruit and nuts on top of the cake.
  Use a pastry brush to brush the glaze over the top of
  the cake.

DATE & PECAN TORTE

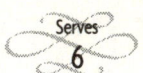
Serves 6

This recipe is a variation of a wicked chocolate, date and nut torte topped with cream and strawberries that my sister Ann introduced to me years ago, but it contains much less fat. You can double the ingredients to make a larger torte. I've tried many topping ideas, but the whipped ricotta cream and lots of fresh strawberries win by a mile.

1 cup dates, finely chopped

1 cup pecans, finely chopped

⅓ cup unbleached white flour

1 teaspoon baking powder

200 g egg whites (about 6 eggs)

½ cup apple juice concentrate

1 teaspoon vanilla essence

1 quantity Ricotta Cream (see page 110)

300 g strawberries, hulled and washed

- Preheat the oven to 160°C. Line a 20 cm round cake tin with baking paper.

- Combine the dates and pecans in a bowl. Sift the flour and baking powder over the top and mix together lightly, taking care to break down any lumps.

- Beat the egg whites until stiff. With the motor running, slowly add the apple juice concentrate and vanilla essence. Gently fold in the dry ingredients.

- Spoon into the prepared tin and bake for 30 minutes or until the top is a light brown and firm to the touch.

- Turn out the torte and cool on a cake rack.

- When cool, spread the ricotta cream over the torte and top with strawberries.

FESTIVE FRUIT & NUT CAKE

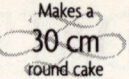

Makes a
30 cm
round cake

There is only one way to eat this cake – in a big warm wedge, straight from the oven! However, if you can hold off, it is just as good cold. It makes an ideal gift for Christmas, wrapped in cellophane with a big tartan bow.

200 g tender dried figs, halved

200 g dried apricots, halved

200 g dates, halved

200 g currants

200 g sultanas

1 tablespoon finely grated orange zest

1 teaspoon mixed spice

½ cup dry sherry

½ cup freshly squeezed orange juice

2 × 425 g cans unsweetened pie
   apples, finely chopped

½ cup apple juice concentrate

200 g egg whites (about 6 eggs)

2 cups unbleached self-raising flour

2 cups unbleached plain flour

300 g mixed nuts (almonds, brazil nuts,
   pecans, hazelnuts)

GLAZE

1 tablespoon brandy, sherry or rum

1 cup Cake and Flan Glaze (see
   page 109)

- Combine the figs, apricots, dates, currants, sultanas, orange zest, mixed spice, sherry, orange juice and apples in a large bowl. Cover and stand overnight.

- Preheat the oven to 150°C. Line a 30 cm round cake tin with a double layer of baking paper.

- Add the apple juice concentrate to the fruit mixture, stirring well.

- Beat the egg whites until stiff. Sift the flours together.

- Add the sifted flour and egg whites to the fruit mixture in alternate lots until all the ingredients are well combined.

- Spoon evenly into the prepared tin. Decorate the top of the cake in a circular pattern with the nuts.

- Bake for 2–2½ hours or until a wooden skewer inserted into the centre of the cake comes out clean.

- Remove from the oven, cover with a tea towel and allow to cool in the tin.

- To make the Glaze, add your preferred liqueur to the cake and flan glaze and cook as described on page 109. Use a pastry brush to spread the glaze evenly over the top of the cake.

FIJI CAKE

One of the most enduring memories of a family Fijian holiday is a chocolate-like cake filled with a whipped, creamy filling of fresh mango and banana pieces. This is my attempt to recapture some of the magical moments.

1 cup unbleached self-raising flour

½ cup unbleached wholemeal self-raising flour

3 tablespoons carob powder

1 teaspoon cinnamon

1 teaspoon mixed spice

1 × 440 g can crushed unsweetened pineapple

½ cup apple juice concentrate

½ cup grapeseed oil

4 egg whites

icing sugar for dusting

FRUIT FILLING

2 × 130 g tub low-fat vanilla frûche

1 mango, peeled and diced

1 banana, peeled and diced

- Preheat the oven to 180°C. Line the base and sides of a 20 cm round cake tin with baking paper.

- Sift the flours, carob powder and spices together.

- Combine the pineapple, pineapple juice, apple juice concentrate and grapeseed oil. Gently fold in the flour.

- Beat the egg whites until stiff and gently fold through the mixture.

- Spoon into the prepared tin and bake for 45 minutes.

- While the cake is baking, make the Fruit Filling by combining all the ingredients. Refrigerate until ready to use.

- Turn out the cake and cool on a wire rack. Cut the cooled cake in half and fill with the fruit filling. Dust the top lightly with icing sugar and serve.

LEMON POPPYSEED RING CAKE

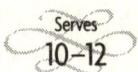
Serves
10–12

This cake is delicious served hot or cold with Lemon Sauce (see page 101) or Orange Citrus Sauce (see page 103), garnished with slices of fresh mango.

1 tablespoon poppyseeds

grated zest of a lemon

2 cups unbleached self-raising flour,
   sifted

$\frac{1}{2}$ cup grapeseed oil

$\frac{1}{2}$ cup apple juice concentrate

$\frac{1}{2}$ cup lemon juice

$\frac{1}{2}$ cup low-fat yoghurt

4 egg whites

- Preheat the oven to 180°C. Line the base of a 25 cm ring tin with baking paper and lightly grease the sides.

- Fold the poppyseeds and lemon zest into the flour.

- Lightly whisk together grapeseed oil, apple juice concentrate and lemon juice. Gradually stir in the flour and poppyseed mixture.

- Fold in the yoghurt.

- Beat the egg whites until stiff and gently fold into the mixture.

- Spoon into the prepared tin and bake for 45 minutes.

- Allow the cake to cool slightly in the tin before turning out onto a cake rack.

PUMPKIN & PRUNE SPICE CAKE

Serves
10–12

This cake is delicious warm or cold. I like it best served with yoghurt
and garnished with grated lemon zest and a sprinkling of nutmeg.

500 g pumpkin, peeled and chopped

1½ cups unbleached self-raising flour

½ cup unbleached wholemeal flour

1 teaspoon cinnamon

1 teaspoon mixed spice

½ teaspoon nutmeg

½ teaspoon ground ginger

200 g prunes, pitted

1 cup low-fat milk or soymilk

½ cup apple juice concentrate

¼ cup grapeseed oil

1 tablespoon bourbon or rum

1 egg

2 egg whites

icing sugar for dusting

- Steam the pumpkin until tender. Drain, mash and leave to cool.

- Preheat the oven to 180°C. Line the base and sides of a rectangular 23 cm loaf tin with baking paper.

- Sift the flours and spices together. Add the prunes.

- Combine the milk, apple juice concentrate, grapeseed oil, bourbon or rum and gently fold in the flour.

- Beat the egg and egg whites together lightly and gently fold into the mixture.

- Spoon into the prepared tin and bake for 45 minutes.

- Turn out the cake and cool on a cake rack. Dust lightly with icing sugar and serve.

FRUIT, GLORIOUS FRUIT

Sometimes the finest desserts are those prepared with the least amount of fuss, using the best and freshest ingredients. A sensational fruit salad, for example, relies on luscious and ripe seasonal fruits. It's best to combine just a few fruits that complement each other rather than mix many different fruits together, so that the subtle flavours don't get lost.

Baked fruits should be poached slowly and gently in just a little water, fruit juice, dessert wine and perhaps a small amount of your favourite liqueur. Baked fruits do not need a lot of added sugar; fruit that is ripe should be sweet enough.

For a warm fruit dessert, baked fruits and even fresh fruits can be wrapped in a parcel using thin layers of filo pastry or topped with a crumble mixture of rolled oats and almonds, and baked in the oven until golden brown. Strudels can be cooked ahead of time and reheated for about 10–15 minutes before serving.

APPLE, BANANA & PINEAPPLE STRUDEL

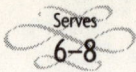

8 sheets filo pastry

3 tablespoons apple juice concentrate

4 tablespoons water

½ cup wholemeal breadcrumbs, toasted

¼ teaspoon cinnamon

600 g cooked apples, well drained and chopped

2 bananas, peeled and sliced

1 × 425 g can unsweetened crushed pineapple, well drained and juices reserved

¼ cup flaked almonds

PINEAPPLE SAUCE

1 cup reserved pineapple juices

1 tablespoon cornflour

- Preheat the oven to 180°C. Cover a baking tray with a sheet of baking paper.

- Place the filo pastry on a slightly damp tea towel and cover with another tea towel or plastic wrap so that the pastry does not dry out while you're working.

- Combine the apple juice concentrate and water.

- Place a sheet of filo on the baking paper and brush with a little of the diluted apple juice concentrate. Place another sheet of pastry on top and repeat until all the pastry is used up.

- Combine the breadcrumbs and cinnamon and spread over base of the pastry where you will place the filling.

- Place the apple down the centre of the pastry, leaving about 5 cm at each end. Top with the banana and the pineapple.

- Fold in 2 cm of the ends, then take the end nearest to you and lift it over the apple mixture. Brush a little of the diluted apple concentrate over the top. Lift up the side of the pastry furthest from you and press down lightly. Do not stretch the pastry over the filling too tightly or the filling will burst through the pastry during cooking.

- Brush the top of the strudel with a little more of the diluted apple juice and sprinkle the top with flaked almonds.

- Bake for 20–30 minutes or until the strudel is golden brown and crisp. Serve with the Pineapple Sauce.

- To make the Pineapple Sauce, mix a little of the pineapple juice with the cornflour to make a paste. Place the remaining pineapple juice in a saucepan. Add the cornflour mixture and stir continuously until the sauce boils and thickens.

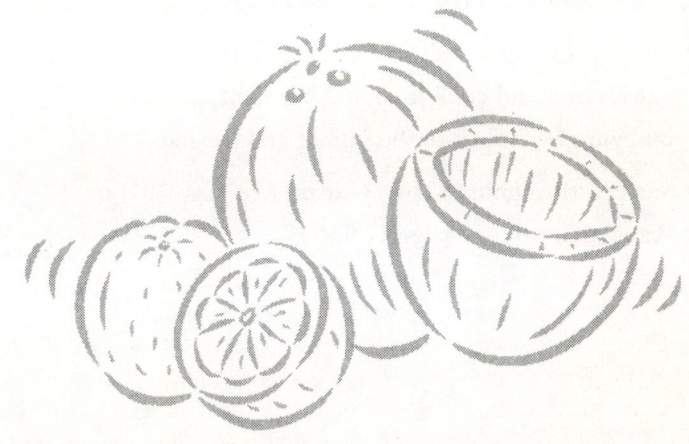

APPLE DUMPLINGS

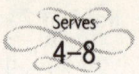

Serves
4–8

This simple recipe is an adaptation of traditional golden syrup dumplings, but without the golden syrup, butter, sugar and eggs. My family agrees that it tastes sensational. You can substitute the apple with other fruits like bananas, pears, apricots and peaches.

SAUCE

1 cup freshly squeezed orange juice

¼ cup water

grated zest of a lemon

½ cup apple juice concentrate

DUMPLINGS

1¼ cups unbleached self-raising flour

1 Granny Smith apple, peeled, cored
  and finely diced

2 egg whites, lightly beaten

½ cup milk

- To make the Sauce, place all the ingredients in a saucepan and bring to a gentle simmer.

- To make the Dumplings, sift the flour into a bowl. Add the diced apple.

- Mix the egg whites and milk together and stir into the flour mixture to make a fairly stiff dough.

- Drop 8 large spoonfuls of the dough into the simmering sauce, cover and cook for about 10 minutes. The dumplings will float to the surface and expand.

- Serve with yoghurt, Citrus Custard (see page 101) or Ricotta Cream (see page 110).

APPLE OAT CRUMBLE

Serves
6

A delicious apple dessert topped with the goodness of rolled oats – perfect for cold winter nights.

6–8 Granny Smith apples, peeled,
  cored and quartered
1 cup unsweetened orange or
  pineapple juice or *freshly squeezed*
  orange juice
1 tablespoon cornflour
grated zest of a lemon

CRUMBLE TOPPING
100 g rolled oats
100 g almonds
4 egg whites
1 teaspoon vanilla essence
2 tablespoons apple juice concentrate

- Gently poach the apples in fruit juice over low heat until just tender. Drain the cooking juices into a saucepan and top up with enough water to make up one cup of liquid.

- Blend the cornflour with enough cold water to make a paste and add to the liquid in the pan with the lemon zest. Stir the mixture over a medium heat until the sauce thickens.

- Place the apples in a shallow baking dish, pour over the sauce and leave to cool and set.

- Preheat the oven to 180°C.

- To make the Crumble Topping, process the rolled oats and almonds until they resemble breadcrumbs.

- Beat the egg whites in a bowl until stiff and slowly add the vanilla essence and apple juice concentrate.

- Fold in the oats and almond mixture and spread evenly over the apples.

- Cook until the top is brown and crunchy. Serve with Basic Custard (see page 99) or ice-cream.

APPLE STRUDEL

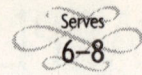

Serves
6-8

Commercially prepared filo pastry has made strudel-making very easy. You simply wrap your favourite fruit and spices or a combination of fruits in layers of the light pastry and bake. Filo pastry is ideal for low-fat desserts because it is made from only flour and water. Traditional strudel recipes call for melted butter to be brushed between the layers of pastry but you can get the same crispy effect by combining a little apple juice concentrate and water. This is a basic recipe; fruits like apricots, peaches, pears or nectarines can be substituted for the apple.

8 sheets filo pastry

3 tablespoons apple juice concentrate

4 tablespoons water

800 g cooked Granny Smith apples,
   well drained and chopped

2 teaspoons grated orange zest

2 teaspoons grated lemon zest

¼ teaspoon cinnamon

¼ teaspoon mixed spice

extra cinnamon

- Preheat the oven to 180°C. Cover a baking tray with a sheet of baking paper.

- Place the filo pastry on a slightly damp tea towel and cover with another tea towel or plastic wrap so that the pastry does not dry out while you're working.

- Combine the apple juice concentrate and water.

- Place a sheet of filo on the baking paper and brush with a little of the diluted apple juice concentrate. Place another sheet of pastry on top and repeat until all the pastry is used up.

- Combine the apple, orange and lemon zest and spices and spoon the mixture into the centre of the pastry, leaving about 5 cm at each end. Fold in 2 cm of the ends, then take the end nearest to you and lift it over the apple mixture. Brush a little of the diluted apple concentrate over the top. Lift up the side of the pastry furthest from you and press down lightly. Do not stretch the pastry over the filling too tightly or the filling will burst through the pastry during cooking.

- Brush the top of the strudel with a little more of the apple juice concentrate and sprinkle liberally with cinnamon.

- Bake for 20–30 minutes or until the strudel is golden brown and crisp. Serve with warm Basic Custard (see page 99) or Orange Citrus Sauce (see page 103).

AUTUMN PEARS

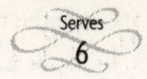

Serves
6

6 ripe but firm pears (Comice or
    Williams or Bartlett pears are ideal)
2 cups unsweetened dark grape juice
2 tablespoons rum or port

peel of 2 oranges
2 teaspoons cornflour
¼ cup water

- Peel the pears, leaving just a little skin around the base and stem.

- Place the pears upright in a saucepan with a fitting lid, pour over the juice and rum or port.

- Remove the peel from the oranges in long thin strips and add to the pan.

- Cover the pears and gently poach until the pears are tender, about 15–20 minutes.

- Remove the pears from the heat and let them stand for at least an hour to absorb the flavour and colour of the juice. You can speed up the process by spooning the juices over the pears every 10 minutes.

- Place the pears on individual serving dishes or a serving platter.

- Combine the cornflour and water. Add to the pear juices in the saucepan and cook, stirring continuously, until the sauce boils and thickens.

- Spoon the sauce over the pears and serve.

BAKED APPLE WITH FRUIT FILLING

Serves 4

This is a favourite dessert for cold nights or winter Sunday afternoons, served with warm Citrus Custard (see page 101).

4 Granny Smith apples	¼ cup lemon juice
60 g mixed dried fruit, finely chopped	¾ cup freshly squeezed orange juice
½ teaspoon ground cinnamon	1 tablespoon apple juice concentrate
½ teaspoon mixed spice	1 teaspoon cornflour
2 teaspoons grated orange zest	1 tablespoon water

- Peel the apples from the stem to halfway down the sides, core and place them in an upright position in a saucepan.

- Combine all the ingredients except for the cornflour and water, and spoon into the apple cores, adding the juices last.

- Cover and gently poach until the apples are tender, about 20–30 minutes. Remove the apples and keep warm.

- Combine the cornflour and water and stir into the cooked apple juices until the sauce boils and thickens. Spoon over the apples.

BANANA & RICOTTA STRUDEL

Serves
4

6–8 sheets filo pastry

2 tablespoons apple juice concentrate

2 tablespoons water

100 g low-fat cottage cheese

150 g ricotta

1 tablespoon apple juice concentrate

¼ teaspoon cinnamon

1 egg

1 egg white

2 bananas, peeled and sliced

½ cup raisins

1 tablespoon finely chopped walnuts

- Preheat the oven to 180°C. Cover a baking tray with a sheet of baking paper.

- Place the filo pastry on a slightly damp tea towel and cover with another tea towel or plastic wrap so that the pastry does not dry out while you're working.

- Combine the apple juice concentrate and water.

- Place a sheet of filo on the baking paper and brush with a little of the diluted apple juice concentrate. Place another sheet of pastry on top and repeat until all the pastry is used up.

- Purée the cottage cheese, ricotta, apple juice concentrate, cinnamon, egg and egg white until smooth and pour the mixture down the centre of the pastry, leaving about 5 cm at each end. Place the banana on top and add the raisins.

- Fold in 2 cm of the ends, then take the end nearest to you and lift it over the apple mixture. Brush a little of the diluted apple concentrate over the top.

- Lift up the side of the pastry furthest from you and press down lightly. Do not stretch the pastry over the filling too tightly or the filling will burst through the pastry during cooking.

- Brush the top with a little more of the apple juice concentrate and sprinkle with walnuts.

- Bake for 20–30 minutes or until the strudel is golden brown and crisp. Serve with Citrus Custard (see page 101) or Orange Citrus Sauce (see page 103).

BANANA FRITTERS

Cinnamon can be substituted for walnuts in this recipe.

2 tablespoons apple juice concentrate   6 bananas, peeled

3 tablespoons water   2 tablespoons finely chopped walnuts

6 sheets filo pastry

- Preheat the oven to 200°C. Cover a baking tray with baking paper. Combine the apple juice concentrate and water.

- Fold each sheet of filo pastry in half and brush with the diluted apple juice.

- Place a whole banana on the pastry, fold over to make a tight parcel and brush well with the diluted apple juice. Roll the parcel in walnuts.

- Repeat with the remaining ingredients.

- Place the bananas on the baking tray, leaving some space between each banana.

- Bake for 10–15 minutes or until the fritters are golden brown.

- Serve with Ricotta Cream (see page 110), ice-cream or yoghurt, or dust lightly with icing sugar and eat immediately.

GINGER PEARS

6 Comice or Bartlett pears

1½ cups unsweetened apple or pear
  juice

½ cup white wine (use a dessert or
  sweet wine)

2 tablespoons glacé ginger, finely
  chopped

2 teaspoons finely grated lemon zest

- Peel the pears, leaving the stems on. Place the pears upright in a saucepan, add the juice, wine, ginger and lemon zest.

- Cover and gently poach until the pears are tender, about 15–20 minutes. Remove the pears and keep warm.

- Bring the pear juices to the boil and reduce by half.

- With a sharp knife, cut the pear from the stem end to the base several times, leaving the slices attached to the stem. Place on individual serving plates and fan out.

- Spoon over some of the ginger sauce. Serve with Citrus Custard (see page 101), yoghurt or Passionfruit Ice-cream (see page 45).

POACHED AMARETTO PEACHES

Serves 8

8 ripe but firm yellow clingstone
  peaches, left whole

2 tablespoons Amaretto liqueur

¼ cup apple juice concentrate

1 cup water

1 teaspoon cornflour

1 tablespoon water

low-fat yoghurt

cinnamon

- Place the peaches, liqueur, apple juice concentrate and water in a shallow pan, cover and gently poach until the peaches are tender, about 10–15 minutes.

- Remove the peaches and keep warm.

- Combine the cornflour and water, add to the peach juices in the pan and cook, stirring continuously, until the sauce boils and thickens. Spoon the sauce over the peaches. Serve with yoghurt and shake over some cinnamon.

- You can also blend the cooked peach juices with some low-fat ricotta to make a delicious creamy sauce.

RED BERRY PASSION FRUIT SALAD

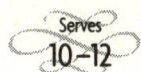

Serves
10–12

Take the freshest fruits in season, toss them in a little fresh juice, perhaps with a little grated citrus zest, or macerate the fruit in a favourite wine or liqueur and you have a delicious fresh fruit salad. Here are two of my favourite recipes. I know you will come up with lots more.

250 g fresh raspberries

200 g blueberries

250 g strawberries

100 g blackberries

250 g mulberries

300 g watermelon, balled

1 tablespoon grated lemon zest

- Mix all the ingredients together and allow to stand for an hour before serving.

TROPICAL PARADISE FRUIT SALAD

Serves
6–8

2 oranges, peeled and diced

1 large mango, peeled and diced

½ pawpaw, peeled, seeds removed
   and diced

½ pineapple, peeled and diced

½ cup passionfruit pulp

- Mix all the ingredients together and allow to stand for an hour before serving.

WINTER FRUIT SALAD

Serves
8–10

Here is a quick-and-easy recipe that maximises the wonderful flavours of dried fruits. You can prepare it ahead of time and keep it in the refrigerator. It can be served with wedges of cantaloupe, sliced oranges or apples, citrus custard, yoghurt or wrapped up in filo pastry for Christmas strudels.

zest from an orange, removed in long, thin strips

100 g dried apricots

100 g dried pears, cut into strips

100 g dried nectarines

1 teaspoon cinnamon

1/4 teaspoon mixed spice

2 cups freshly squeezed orange juice

1/2 cup muscat, brandy or port

100 g fresh dates, stones removed

100 g prunes, stones removed

100 g dried figs

3/4 cup slivered almonds

- Combine the orange zest, apricots, pears, nectarines, cinnamon, mixed spice, orange juice and muscat in a saucepan and gently simmer, uncovered, for 10 minutes.

- Add the dates, prunes and figs, and cook for a further 2 minutes.

- Remove from the heat and fold in the almonds.

- Spoon the mixture into a clean, dry jar.

- Boil the remaining juices until reduced by half and pour into the jar. Seal and refrigerate.

ICE-CREAMS & SORBETS

*W*hether you are young or old, ice-cream and frozen flavoured ice treats are a favourite. However, the commercial varieties tend to be loaded with saturated fats, artificial flavourings, colourings and lots of sugar. The traditional recipes, on the other hand, are usually a combination of cream, egg yolks and again, lots of sugar. So while we may love the taste of ice-creams and sorbets, they are not always practical in a low-fat diet.

The solution is to make your own. It is very easy to make sensational tasting, low-fat ice-creams and delicious sorbets at home, using low-fat ingredients and the natural sweet flavours of fruits that are in season.

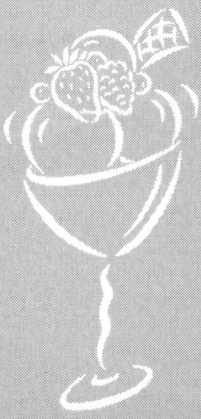

MAKING ICE-CREAM & SORBET

The best results when making ice-cream or sorbet come from an ice-cream machine. If you do not own one, follow these steps for great results every time.

Step 1 All ingredients should be well chilled.

Step 2 Equipment such as metal bowls and spoons should be placed in the freezer for 15 minutes before using.

Step 3 Pour ice-cream or sorbet into a well-chilled metal tray.

Step 4 To prevent the ice-cream or sorbet from becoming too icy in texture, let it nearly set and beat again in a well-chilled bowl until stiff. Return to a very cold freezer.

Step 5 Allow the ice-cream or sorbet to soften slightly in the refrigerator before serving.

Step 6 Low-fat ice-creams and sorbets do not store well and tend to become rock hard the longer they stay in the freezer. Should the ice-cream or sorbet become too hard, place in a food processor and quickly blend to a creamy consistency. Eat immediately.

APRICOT SORBET

Serves
6–8

Banana and passionfruit are perfect accompaniments to this sorbet.

200 g dried apricots   ¼ cup apple juice concentrate

2 cups water   2 teaspoons almond essence

½ cup freshly squeezed orange juice   1 tablespoon grated lemon zest

- Place the apricots in a saucepan, add enough water to just cover and simmer uncovered until the apricots are quite soft. Drain.

- Place the apricots, 2 cups water, orange juice, apple juice concentrate and almond essence in a blender and purée.

- Fold in the lemon zest.

- Pour the mixture into an ice-cream machine and follow the manufacturer's instructions. If you do not have an ice-cream machine, follow the instructions on page 38.

- Spoon the sorbet into tall dessert goblets or champagne flutes.

BOYSENBERRY ICE-CREAM

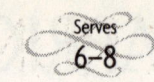

Serves
6–8

This ice-cream is delicious on its own or served with fresh berries. It looks and tastes particularly good served with slices of kiwifruit. You can turn this basic recipe into a gourmet one by adding some finely chopped macadamias, shredded coconut or raisins that have been macerated in a little rum.

1 × 375 ml can evaporated milk *or*	1 teaspoon gelatine
375 ml low-fat soymilk, well chilled	1 tablespoon boiling water
1 teaspoon vanilla essence	400 g boysenberries, fresh or frozen
2 tablespoons apple juice concentrate	

- Beat the milk and vanilla essence until thick, creamy and frothy, and doubled in size. If the mixture does not double in size, it means the ingredients were not chilled enough. Place the mixture in the freezer for 30 minutes and beat again.

- Add the apple juice concentrate to the milk.

- Dissolve the gelatine in boiling water, and add to the mixture.

- Fold in the boysenberries.

- Pour the mixture into an ice-cream machine and churn following the manufacturer's instructions. If you do not have an ice-cream machine, follow the instructions on page 38.

CHUNKY BANANA ICE-CREAM

Serves 8

Serve this ice-cream with slices of mango and pawpaw and spoon over lots of fresh passionfruit pulp . . . delicious!

1 × 375 ml can evaporated skim milk or 375 ml low-fat soymilk, well chilled

3 teaspoons vanilla essence

1 teaspoon gelatine

1 tablespoon boiling water

2 tablespoons lemon juice

1 teaspoon grated orange zest

4 bananas, peeled and chopped

- Beat the milk and vanilla essence until it is thick, creamy and doubled in size. If the mixture does not double in size, it means the ingredients were not chilled enough. Place the mixture in the freezer for 30 minutes and beat again.

- Dissolve the gelatine in boiling water, stir in the lemon juice and add this to the milk mixture.

- Fold in the orange zest and bananas.

- Pour the mixture into an ice-cream machine and churn following the manufacturer's instructions. If you do not have an ice-cream machine, follow the instructions on page 38.

KIWIFRUIT & GINGER SORBET

Serves
6–8

Allow your taste buds to determine the amount of green ginger wine to use.

1 kg kiwifruit, peeled and chopped	1 teaspoon lemon juice
2 tablespoons apple juice concentrate	1 teaspoon finely grated lime zest
¼ cup green ginger wine	

- Purée all the ingredients together.

- Pour the mixture into an ice-cream machine and churn following the manufacturer's instructions. If you do not have an ice-cream machine, follow the instructions on page 38.

- Spoon the sorbet into tall dessert goblets and top with slices of kiwifruit and black and green grapes if you like.

OPPOSITE
Carob & Date Mud Cake (see page 8).

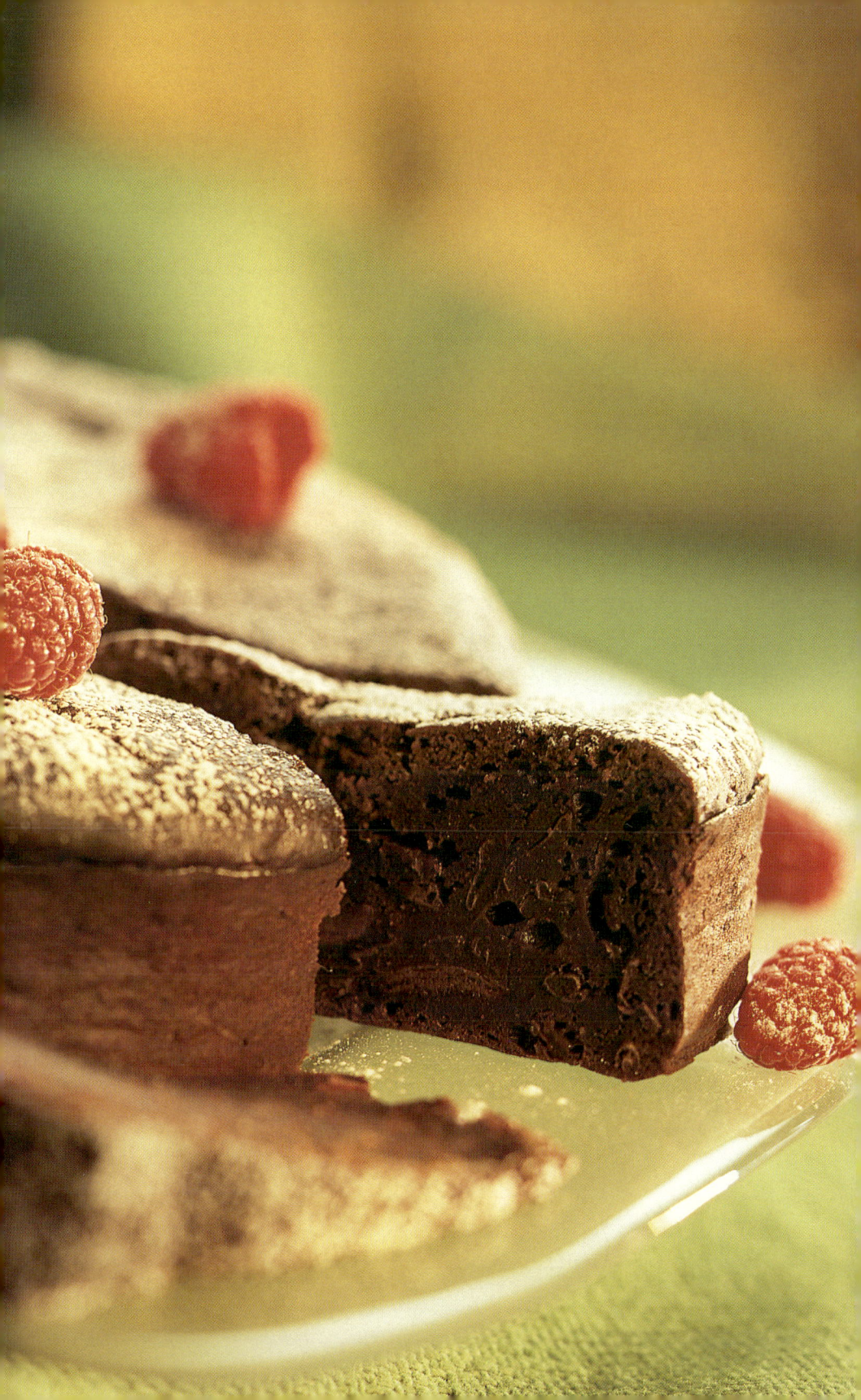

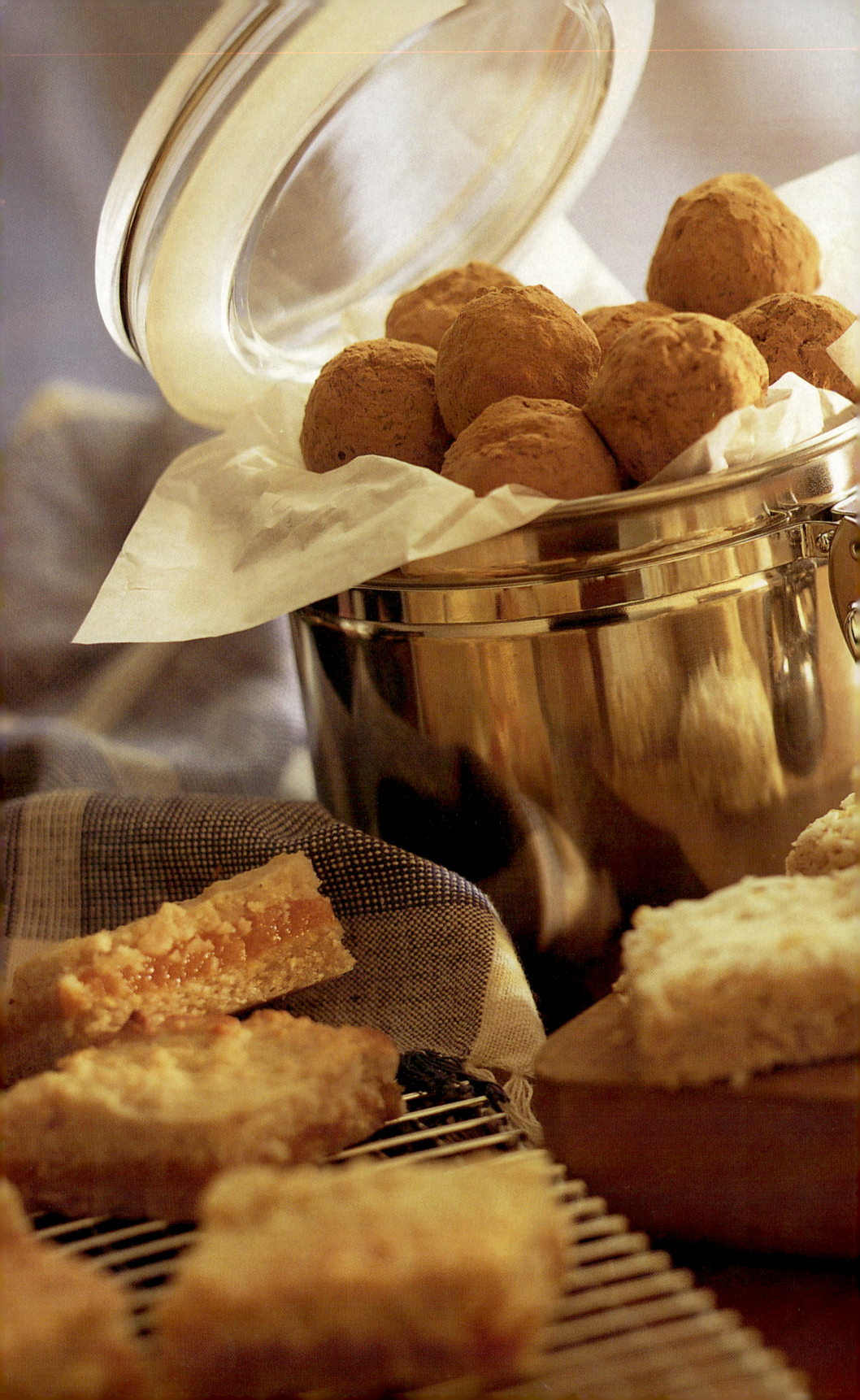

ORANGE, RAISIN & MACADAMIA NUT ICE-CREAM

Serves 6

This ice-cream is particularly good served with fresh orange slices or bananas. The orange zest gives taste as well as colour.

1 × 375 ml evaporated skim milk, well
  chilled
1 teaspoon orange essence
1 tablespoon grated orange zest
¼ cup apple juice concentrate
1 teaspoon gelatine

1 tablespoon boiling water
1 tablespoon freshly squeezed orange
  juice
¼ cup finely chopped raisins
¼ cup finely chopped macadamias

- Beat the milk, orange essence and orange zest until the mixture is thick, creamy and doubled in size. If the mixture does not double in size, it means the ingredients were not chilled enough. Place the mixture in the freezer for 30 minutes and beat again.

- Add the apple juice concentrate.

- Dissolve the gelatine in boiling water, stir in the orange juice and add to the milk mixture. >

OPPOSITE
Carob Hedgehog Balls (see page 9), Apricot Crumble Slice (see page 3), and Chewy Banana & Nut Slice (see page 12).

- Pour the mixture into an ice-cream machine and churn following the manufacturer's instructions. If you do not have an ice-cream machine, follow the instructions on page 38.

- Fold in the raisins and macadamias about 10 minutes into the freezing process. If you do not have an ice-cream machine, add them before you place the ice-cream in the freezer for the first time (see step 4, page 38).

PASSIONFRUIT ICE-CREAM

Serves
8

Passionfruit ice-cream is excellent to serve with warm puddings or cakes.

pulp of 10 passionfruit

1 × 375 ml can evaporated skim milk,
    well chilled

¼ cup apple juice concentrate

1 teaspoon gelatine

1 tablespoon boiling water

2 teaspoons lemon juice

- Strain the passionfruit juice from the pulp. You should have about a cup of juice. Use more passionfruit if necessary.

- Beat the milk until thick, creamy and doubled in size. If it does not double in size, it means the ingredients were not chilled enough. Place the mixture in the freezer for 30 minutes and beat again.

- Slowly add the passionfruit juice and apple juice concentrate.

- Dissolve the gelatine in boiling water, add the lemon juice and add to the milk mixture.

- You can stir a teaspoon or more of the passionfruit seeds into the ice-cream at this stage for visual effect.

- Pour the mixture into an ice-cream machine and churn following the manufacturer's instructions. If you do not have an ice-cream machine, follow the instructions on page 38.

PEAR *&* LEMON SORBET

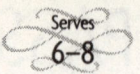

Serves
6–8

1 × 850 g can unsweetened pears   *¼ cup lemon juice*
¼ cup apple juice concentrate   *1 teaspoon grated lemon zest*

- Push the pears through a strainer to make a purée. Stir in the pear juice, apple juice concentrate, lemon juice and zest.

- Pour the mixture into an ice-cream machine and churn following the manufacturer's instructions. If you do not have an ice-cream machine, follow the instructions on page 38.

- Spoon the sorbet into tall dessert goblets or champagne flutes and garnish with some fresh mint leaves.

PINEAPPLE & MANGO ICE-CREAM

Serves
8

A good recipe to make when mangoes are plentiful and cheap.

1 × 375 ml can evaporated skim milk,
 well chilled

1 teaspoon orange essence

1 × 425 g can unsweetened crushed
 pineapple

1 mango, peeled and finely chopped

1 teaspoon grated orange zest

¼ cup apple juice concentrate

1 teaspoon gelatine

1 tablespoon boiling water

1 tablespoon lemon juice

- Beat the milk and orange essence until thick, creamy and doubled in size. If the mixture does not double in size, it means the ingredients were not chilled enough. Place the mixture in the freezer for 30 minutes and beat again.

- Slowly add the crushed pineapple, pineapple juice, mango, orange zest and apple juice concentrate.

- Dissolve the gelatine in boiling water, add the lemon juice and add to the milk mixture.

- Pour the mixture into an ice-cream machine and churn following the manufacturer's instructions. If you do not have an ice-cream machine, follow the instructions on page 38.

RICH CREAM CAROB & COCONUT ICE-CREAM

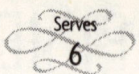

Serves 6

Serve with fresh strawberries or raspberry sauce.

1 × 375 ml can evaporated skim milk, well chilled

¼ cup coconut milk, well chilled

2–3 tablespoons carob powder

1 tablespoon rum

2 teaspoons vanilla essence

¼ cup boiling water

¼ cup apple juice concentrate

2 teaspoons gelatine

2 tablespoons boiling water

- Beat the milk until thick, creamy and doubled in size. If the mixture does not double in size, it means the ingredients were not chilled enough. Place the mixture in the freezer for 30 minutes and beat again.

- With the motor running, slowly add the coconut milk.

- Combine the carob powder, rum, vanilla essence and boiling water and mix to make a paste.

- Add the apple juice concentrate to the carob mixture, and fold into the milk mixture.

- Dissolve the gelatine in boiling water and add to the milk mixture.

- Pour the mixture into an ice-cream machine and churn following the manufacturer's instructions. If you do not have an ice-cream machine, follow the instructions on page 38.

STRAWBERRY ICE-CREAM

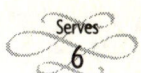

Serves
6

Delicious served with fresh fruit or in a sugar-free ice-cream cone.

1 × 375 ml can evaporated skim milk,
  well chilled

2 teaspoons vanilla essence

2 tablespoons apple juice concentrate

500 g strawberries, hulled and
  chopped

1 teaspoon gelatine

2 tablespoons boiling water

2 tablespoons freshly squeezed
  orange juice

- Beat the milk and vanilla essence until thick, creamy and doubled in size. If the mixture does not double in size, it means the ingredients were not chilled enough. Place the mixture in the freezer for 30 minutes and beat again.

- Slowly add the apple juice concentrate.

- Reserve 1 cup of the strawberries and fold the remaining ones into the milk mixture.

- Dissolve the gelatine in boiling water, stir in the orange juice and add to the milk mixture.

- Pour the mixture into an ice-cream machine and churn following the manufacturer's instructions. If you do not have an ice-cream machine, follow the instructions on page 38.

- Fold in the remaining strawberries 15 minutes into the freezing process. If you do not have an ice-cream machine, add them before you place the ice-cream in the freezer for the first time (see step 4, page 38).

WATERMELON & APPLE SPICE SORBET

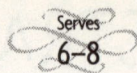

Serves
6–8

600 g watermelon flesh

1 × 850 g can unsweetened pie apple

½–1 teaspoon mixed spice

1 tablespoon lime juice

2 teaspoons grated lemon or
orange zest

- Push the watermelon flesh through a strainer and discard the seeds.

- Purée the apple and stir in the watermelon juice, mixed spice, lime juice and lemon zest.

- Pour the mixture into an ice-cream machine and churn following the manufacturer's instructions. If you do not have an ice-cream machine, follow the instructions on page 38.

- Spoon the sorbet into tall dessert goblets, champagne flutes or cut the tops off red or green apples, scoop out the flesh and fill with sorbet. Garnish with some fresh berries and strawberry leaves if you like.

MOUSSES, JELLIES & FRUIT SWIRLS

These desserts fit into the category of quick-and-easy, soft sweets that bring together the wonderful flavours and colours of fresh or lightly poached fruits with low-fat yoghurt, a light, low-fat custard or a fruit sauce. You can take these desserts from being visually ordinary to stunning in the way you present them. Find some tall parfait or champagne flutes, a stunning glass bowl, attractive shaped moulds or a long terrine dish and create layers with the ingredients, or swirl them together to create ripple effects. To finish, perhaps a light dusting of icing sugar, a fresh peppermint leaf, berries or finely diced fresh fruit as garnish – your family and friends will be impressed.

APRICOT & PASSIONFRUIT MOUSSE

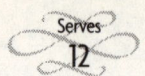

Serves
12

20 dried apricots

¼ cup freshly squeezed orange juice

1 × 375 ml can evaporated skim milk, well chilled

1 teaspoon vanilla essence

1 tablespoon apple juice concentrate

1 teaspoon white wine vinegar

1 tablespoon gelatine

¼ cup boiling water

1 quantity Ricotta Cream (see page 110)

¼ cup passionfruit pulp

- Simmer the apricots in ½ cup of the orange juice until they are soft. Purée.

- Beat the milk until thick, creamy and doubled in size and, while stirring, add the apricot mixture, vanilla essence, apple juice concentrate and vinegar.

- Dissolve the gelatine in boiling water, add the remaining orange juice and fold into the mousse mixture.

- Pour the mixture into a mould and refrigerate until firm.

- Top with ricotta cream and passionfruit pulp just before serving.

BAKED COCONUT CUSTARD

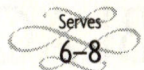

Serves
6–8

SAUCE

½ cup freshly squeezed orange juice

¼ cup apple juice concentrate

CUSTARD

3 cups low-fat milk or soymilk

½ cup coconut milk powder

2 eggs

2 egg whites

1 tablespoon apple juice concentrate

1 tablespoon vanilla essence

- Preheat the oven to 180°C.

- Mix the Sauce ingredients together in a saucepan and bring to the boil.

- Purée all the Custard ingredients.

- Pour the boiling sauce into the base of a baking dish. Pour over the custard.

- Place the baking dish into a tray filled with enough warm water to reach halfway up the sides of the dish.

- Bake for 40 minutes or until the custard is firm.

- Allow the custard to stand for 30 minutes before serving or refrigerate and serve the custard cold.

BLACKBERRY & APPLE FRUIT SWIRLS

200 g low-fat cottage cheese   ¼ teaspoon cinnamon

250 g low-fat ricotta   3 cups blackberries

2 tablespoons apple juice concentrate   2 cups cooked apple, well drained

- Purée the cottage cheese, ricotta, apple juice concentrate and cinnamon until smooth and creamy.

- Place some blackberries at the base of each dessert goblet, top with some of the creamy mixture, add some apple, top with more blackberries and the creamy mixture. Save some blackberries to decorate the top of each goblet. Chill before serving.

BLUEBERRY YOGHURT FRUIT SWIRLS

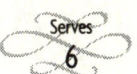

1 quantity Blueberry Sauce (see
   page 100)
2 ½ cups low-fat yoghurt

1 tablespoon finely chopped pecans
2 tablespoons toasted shredded
   coconut

- Add the blueberry sauce to the yoghurt and stir lightly to create a swirl effect.

- Combine the pecans and coconut.

- Spoon the mixture into dessert goblets and garnish each with a little of the pecan and coconut mixture. Chill before serving.

CAROB MOUSSE

4 cups low-fat milk

1 cup cornflour

2 teaspoons vanilla essence

¼ cup apple juice concentrate

2 tablespoons carob or cocoa powder

¼ cup boiling water

1 tablespoon grated orange zest

1 cup low-fat yoghurt

4 egg whites

icing sugar for dusting

- Mix some of the milk with the cornflour to make a paste.

- Place the remaining milk, vanilla essence and apple juice concentrate in a saucepan, stir in the cornflour mixture, and slowly bring to the boil, stirring continuously until the mixture thickens.

- While the mixture is cooking, combine the carob or cocoa with boiling water, stir to dissolve, and add to the mixture. Add the orange zest.

- Remove the mixture from the heat and allow to cool a little before folding in the yoghurt.

- Beat the egg whites until stiff and gently fold into the mixture.

- Pour into a mould or individual moulds and refrigerate until firm.

- Dust with a little icing sugar and serve with strawberries.

JELLIED FRUIT SALAD

200 g pineapple, peeled and finely
  chopped

100 g strawberries, hulled and halved

100 g peaches, peeled and finely
  chopped

100 g kiwifruit, peeled and finely
  chopped

50 g orange, peeled, pith removed and
  finely chopped

50 g mango, peeled and finely
  chopped

2–3 tablespoons apple juice
  concentrate

2 cups water

2 teaspoons agar powder

- Collect all the fruit juices that result from chopping the fruits.

- Place the apple juice concentrate, water and agar powder in a saucepan and slowly bring to the boil, stirring continuously until the agar is dissolved.

- Fold in the fruit and reserved fruit juices. Pour the mixture into a mould and refrigerate until firm.

- The fruit mould can be served with yoghurt, Basic Custard (see page 99) or ice-cream.

LEMON MOUSSE

Serves
6

1 cup evaporated skim milk, well
   chilled

1 teaspoon gelatine

2 tablespoons boiling water

2 tablespoons freshly squeezed orange
   juice

1 cup cold Lemon Sauce (see page 101)

- Beat the milk until thick, creamy and doubled in size.

- Dissolve the gelatine in boiling water, add the orange
  juice and fold into the milk mixture.

- Add the lemon sauce and continue beating until well
  combined. Pour the mixture into a mould or dessert
  goblets and refrigerate until firm.

PASSIONFRUIT &
LEMON SWIRLS

Serves
6

3 cups low-fat fromage frais or
   low-fat yoghurt

1 quantity Lemon Sauce (see page 101)

pulp of 6 passionfruit

- Mix a cup of the fromage frais or yoghurt with a cup of
  lemon sauce.

- Spoon alternate layers of fromage frais, the lemon
  mixture and passionfruit pulp into dessert goblets,
  finishing with the passionfruit pulp. Chill before serving.

OPPOSITE
Autumn Pears (see page 28).

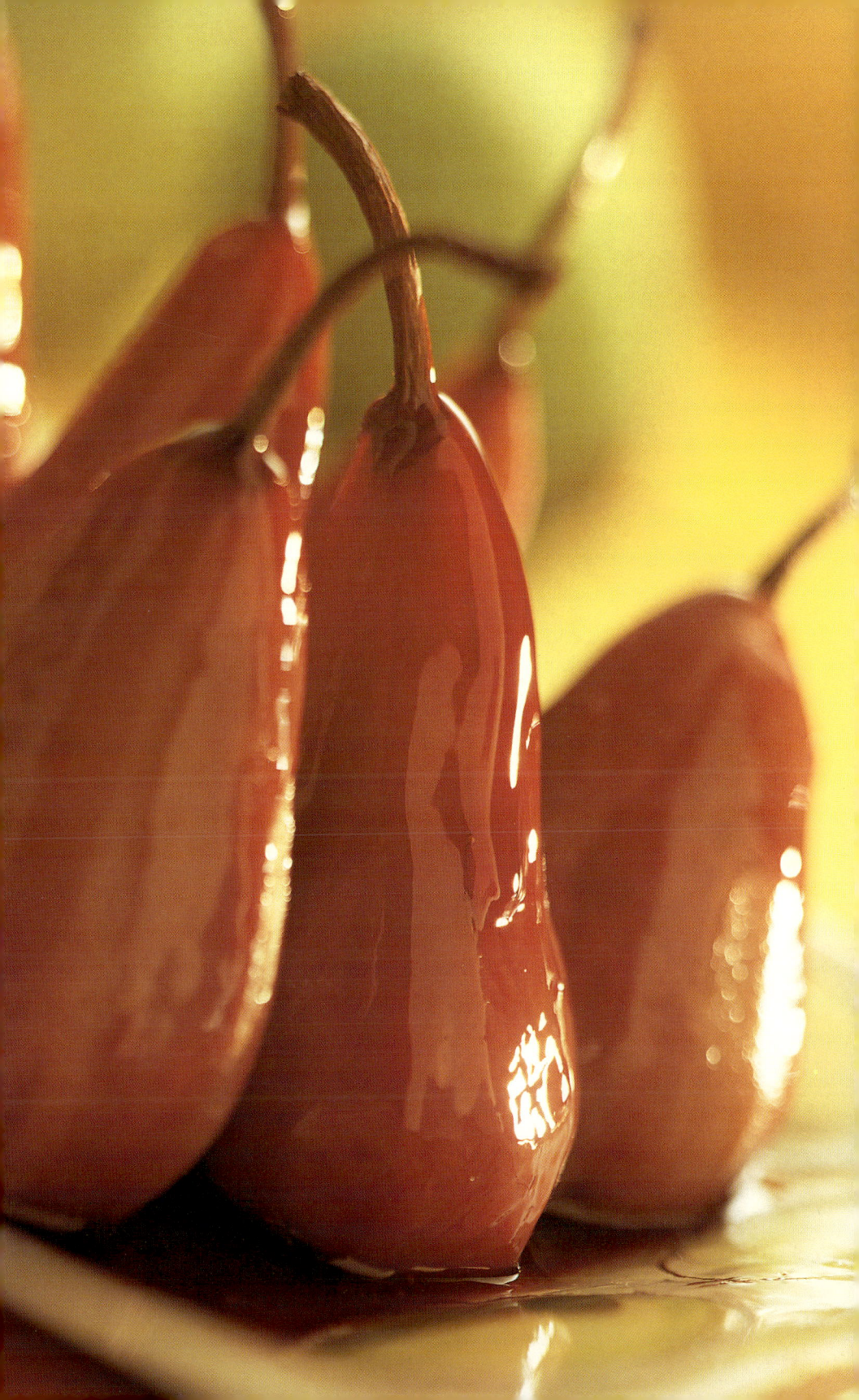

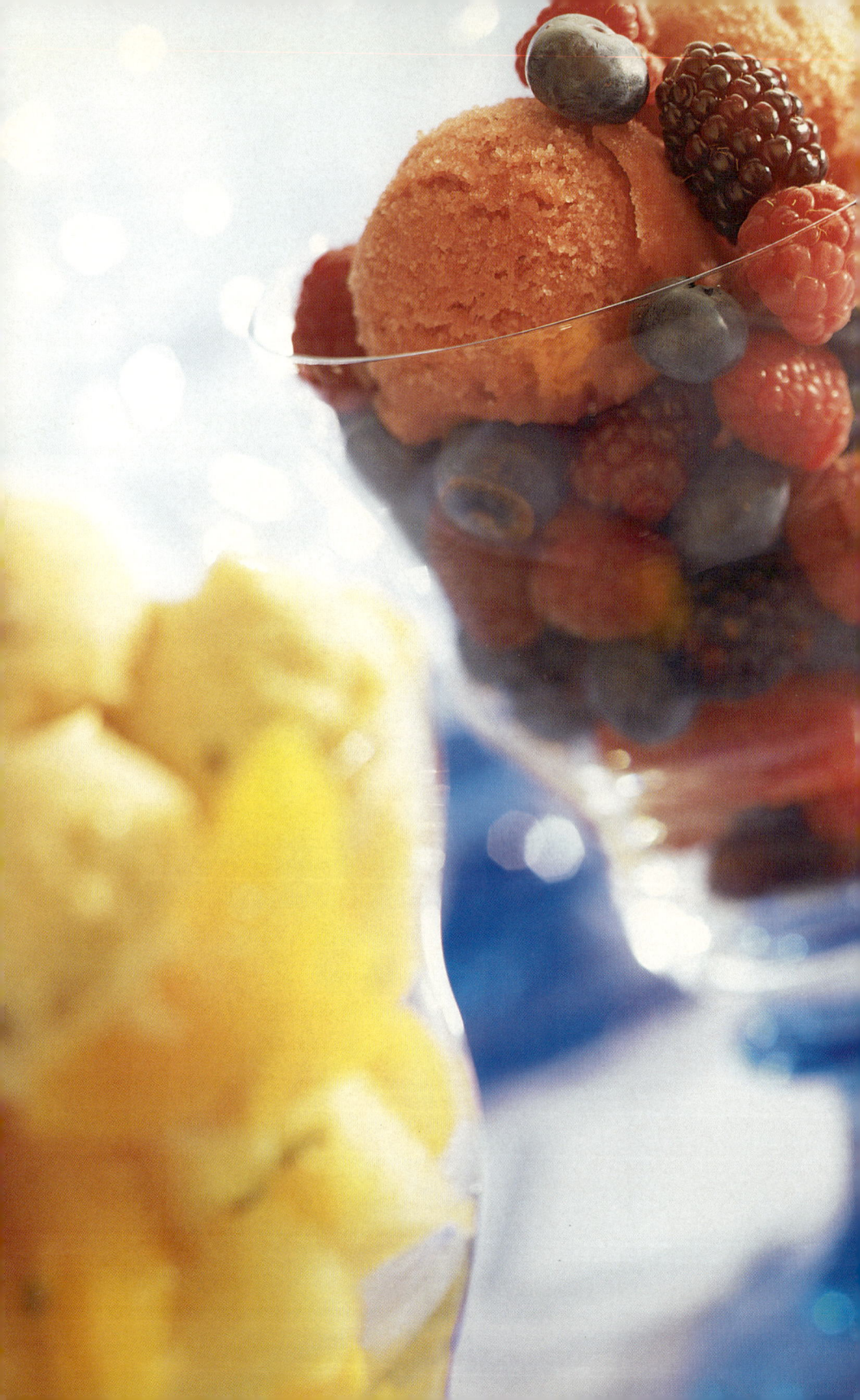

PEACH & YOGHURT MOUSSE

Serves
6–8

1 × 825 g can unsweetened peaches,
    well drained

2 tablespoons apple juice concentrate

2 teaspoons almond essence

1 tablespoon gelatine

¼ cup boiling water

1 tablespoon lemon juice

1½ cups low-fat yoghurt

- Purée the peaches, apple juice concentrate and almond essence.

- Dissolve the gelatine in boiling water, add the lemon juice and fold into the peach mixture.

- Fold in the yoghurt.

- Pour the mixture into a mould or dessert goblets and refrigerate until firm.

- This mousse is perfect to serve with fresh mango, pawpaw, pineapple, passionfruit, Raspberry Sauce (see page 104) or Winter Fruit Salad (see page 36).

OPPOSITE

Watermelon & Apple Spice Sorbet (see page 50)
with Red Berry Passion Fruit Salad (see page 35),
and Passionfruit Ice-cream (see page 45).

RASPBERRY & WALNUT FRUIT SWIRLS

Serves
4

2 cups Basic Custard (see page 99)

1 quantity Raspberry Sauce (see
   page 104)

1 cup fresh raspberries

2 tablespoons finely chopped walnuts

icing sugar for dusting

- Pour alternate layers of custard and raspberry sauce into dessert goblets.

- Decorate with the raspberries and walnuts and dust lightly with icing sugar. Chill before serving.

RASPBERRY MOUSSE

Serves
6

1 cup evaporated skim milk, well
   chilled

1 teaspoon vanilla essence

½ teaspoon cinnamon

1 tablespoon gelatine

¼ cup boiling water

2 tablespoons freshly squeezed orange
   juice

1 cup raspberries, fresh or frozen

1 tablespoon apple juice concentrate

- Beat the milk, vanilla and cinnamon until thick, creamy and doubled in size.

- Dissolve the gelatine in boiling water, add the orange juice and fold into the milk mixture.

- Add the raspberries and apple juice concentrate.

- Pour the mixture into a mould or dessert goblets and refrigerate until firm.

PIES & PUDDINGS

In this section you'll find puddings and pies that can be served hot or cold. All of these desserts are quite substantial in themselves, and should follow a light main meal. You may like to serve slightly larger portions as a sweet main meal. One of my favourites here is Banana Yoghurt Pie, which is an adaption of a very rich dessert I sampled on my first visit to America. This recipe has far less kilojoules and fat, uses carob as an alternative to chocolate, and tastes even better than the original.

Cold Christmas Pudding is a dessert I came up with one Christmas when it was just too hot to serve up the traditional hot Christmas pudding. It has now become a favourite and is made throughout the year. The bread puddings, without the usual butter, make delicious wholesome desserts for the middle of winter. During summer I can't seem to go past finding every possible excuse to make yet another berry pudding while the berries are still in season.

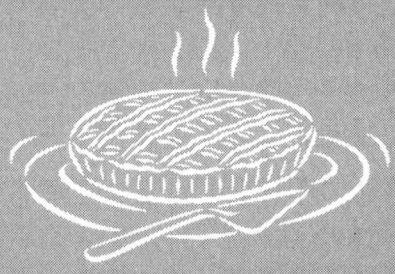

APPLE & GINGER PIE

Serves
8–10

1 quantity Cinnamon Pastry (see
  page 106)
2 tablespoons apple juice
  concentrate
2 tablespoons water

FILLING
1.5 kg Granny Smith apples, peeled,
  cored and thinly sliced
225 g glacé ginger, finely chopped
1 tablespoon lemon juice
1 tablespoon finely grated orange zest

- To make the Filling, place the apples in a saucepan and
  cover with water. Cover and gently poach until soft.
  Add the ginger, lemon juice and orange zest and allow
  to stand until cool.

- Preheat the oven to 180°C. Lightly grease a pie dish.

- Divide the pastry into two equal lots. Roll out each lot
  of pastry separately to fit the base and top of the dish.

- Press the bottom half over the base of the prepared dish
  and spread the cooled filling over the base.

- Combine the apple juice concentrate and water.

- Top with the pastry lid and squeeze the edges together.
  If there is any leftover pastry you can use this to decorate
  the top of pie. Brush a little of the combined apple juice
  concentrate and water over the areas where you want
  pastry to stick. Cut some small holes in the top of the pie
  so that the steam can escape.

- Brush the top of the pie with the combined apple juice
  concentrate and water, then bake for 30–40 minutes or
  until the top is golden brown.

BANANA YOGHURT PIE

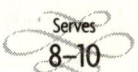

Serves
8–10

A very sweet pie that has American origins. True chocoholics have been known to believe they are devouring a rich chocolate base. A small slice goes a long way. It keeps well — if there's any left over to keep, that is!

BASE

225 g rolled oats

200 g dates, stoned

2 tablespoons carob powder

1 tablespoon vanilla essence

2 tablespoons freshly squeezed orange
    juice

FILLING

¼ cup boiling water

1 tablespoon gelatine

2 frozen bananas, peeled and chopped

250 ml low-fat evaporated milk, well
    chilled

½ teaspoon vanilla essence

250 ml low-fat yoghurt

¼ cup lemon juice

1 fresh banana, finely sliced

1 teaspoon ground nutmeg

- To make the Base, combine the rolled oats, dates and carob powder in a food processor. Process until the mixture resembles breadcrumbs.

- Add the vanilla essence and orange juice and continue to process until the mixture just begins to stick together.

- Lightly grease a shallow 23 cm fluted pie dish.

- Press the pastry thinly and firmly around the sides and base of the dish and refrigerate until the base is quite firm. >

- To make the Filling, pour boiling water over the gelatine, stir to dissolve and set aside to cool.

- Place the frozen bananas in a food processor or blender and blend until smooth.

- Add the milk and blend for a further 3–5 minutes or until the mixture is thick, creamy and doubled in size.

- Add the vanilla essence, yoghurt and gelatine mixture.

- Pour the filling over the base and refrigerate for at least 2–3 hours or until firm.

- Pour the lemon juice over the sliced banana and allow to stand for 10 minutes. Just before serving, garnish the top with banana and sprinkle with nutmeg.

BERRY PUDDING

Serves
8

This is a simple dessert with a memorable flavour that makes you want to go back for seconds. You can double the quantities very easily to make a larger pudding, which looks stunning for special occasions. When you unmould the pudding, scatter lots of fresh raspberries and blueberries over the top and dust lightly with icing sugar.

1 cup water

3 tablespoons apple juice concentrate

½ teaspoon agar powder

1.5 kg mixed berries (blueberries,

raspberries, mulberries), fresh or

frozen

16 slices white high-fibre bread, crusts

removed

- Place the water, apple juice concentrate and agar powder in a saucepan and slowly bring to the boil, stirring continuously to dissolve the agar.

- Add the berries, stir and gently cook until the berries begin to release their colour and juices.

- Cut each slice of bread in half. Line a medium-sized pudding basin with the slices, overlapping slightly to make sure there are no gaps.

- Pour a large spoonful of berry juice over the base and allow it to soak into the bread before adding the remaining berry mixture.

- Cover the berries with the remaining bread slices.

- Cover the top of the pudding with plastic wrap. Place a large plate weighted down with a heavy object on top.

- Refrigerate for at least 4–6 hours before slicing. Serve the pudding with extra fresh berries and yoghurt.

BERRY SUMMER JELLY PUDDING

Serves
8

*If you like the flavour of summer's most loved fruits — berries — but
not the bread, here's a recipe that omits it.*

880 g berries (strawberries,   4 cups water
    blueberries, raspberries, red   4 teaspoons agar powder
    currants, cherries)   ¼ cup apple juice concentrate

- Clean the berries, remove any stems, halve the
  strawberries. Remove the pips from the cherries and cut
  in half.

- Place the water, agar and apple juice concentrate in a
  saucepan and slowly bring to the boil, stirring
  continuously to dissolve the agar.

- Add the berries, stirring carefully until the fruits start to
  bleed their colours into the liquid. Do not overcook.

- Remove from the heat and pour the mixture into a
  round pudding bowl. Refrigerate until firm.

- Cut the pudding into wedges and serve with yoghurt,
  ice-cream or sliced kiwifruit.

CHOCOLATE PUDDINGS WITH RASPBERRY SAUCE

Serves 6

1 quantity Raspberry Sauce   *½ cup boiling water*
  (see page 104)   *½ cup apple juice concentrate*
1 cup unbleached self-raising flour   *2 teaspoons vanilla essence*
½ teaspoon bicarbonate of soda   *1 cup low-fat milk*
⅓ cup cocoa or carob powder   *4 egg whites*

- Preheat the oven to 180°C. Lightly grease 6 individual pudding moulds.

- Spoon equal amounts of raspberry sauce into the base of each pudding mould.

- Sift the flour and bicarbonate of soda into a bowl.

- Mix the cocoa or carob and boiling water, stir until smooth, and add the apple juice concentrate, vanilla essence and milk.

- Slowly add the flour to the cocoa mixture and mix well.

- Beat the egg whites until stiff and gently fold into the chocolate mixture.

- Spoon evenly into the pudding moulds and place the moulds onto a baking tray. Fill the tray with enough warm water to reach halfway up the sides of the moulds.

- Bake for 50 minutes or until the centre of the puddings are quite firm.

- Dust with icing sugar and serve with fresh berries (raspberries, blueberries, strawberries).

COLD CHRISTMAS PUDDING

This is an ideal dessert for those hot Christmas days when a heavy Christmas pudding is simply too much to bear. I like to serve it on my biggest glass platter, surrounded with a selection of all the wonderful fruits available at Christmas time. It can be made well ahead of time and refrigerated.

100 g sultanas

100 g dried apricots, finely chopped

100 g prunes, stoned and chopped

100 g currants

1 cup freshly squeezed orange juice

1 teaspoon mixed spice

2 tablespoons dry sherry

1 × 425 g can sliced cooked apple, chopped

1 tablespoon lemon juice

½ cup unsweetened apple juice

2 tablespoons gelatine

¼ cup boiling water

- Combine the dried fruits, orange juice, mixed spice and sherry in a saucepan and slowly bring to the boil. Simmer for about 3 minutes and allow to cool slightly.

- Fold in the apples. Combine the lemon and apple juices.

- Dissolve the gelatine in boiling water and add to the juices. Pour the gelatine mixture into the dried fruit mixture and mix well.

- Spoon into a 1.5-litre pudding mould, cover and refrigerate overnight or even longer.

- Unmould the pudding onto a platter and use a warm, sharp knife to slice into portions.

CREAMY COCONUT & APRICOT RICE PUDDING

Serves
8–10

100 g Arborio short-grain rice	150 g dried apricots, finely chopped
2 cups low-fat milk or soymilk	1 tablespoon finely grated lemon zest
1 cup coconut milk	4 egg whites
2 tablespoons apple juice concentrate	icing sugar for dusting

- Place the rice and low-fat milk in a large heavy-based saucepan, stir thoroughly, cover and very slowly heat the milk and rice. The milk should not boil, but simmer gently. Allow to simmer for 15 minutes, then remove from the heat. Stir once or twice during the cooking time and allow the rice to stand until it is soft.

- Add the coconut milk, apple juice concentrate, apricots and lemon zest.

- Preheat the oven to 170°C. Lightly grease a shallow baking dish.

- Beat the egg whites until stiff and gently fold into the rice mixture.

- Pour the rice mixture into the prepared dish and bake for 30–35 minutes.

- Dust lightly with icing sugar and serve warm or cold.

LEMON MERINGUE PIE

This alternative to the traditional lemon meringue pie is much healthier, and has just as much lemony flavour. The crunchy topping is quite a surprise.

1 quantity Sweet Pastry (see page 107)
  or ½ quantity Wholemeal Pecan
  Pastry (see page 108)

1¼ cups water
½ cup cornflour

FILLING
¾ cup lemon juice
½ cup apple juice concentrate
1 tablespoon grated orange zest
1 tablespoon grated lemon zest

MERINGUE
4 egg whites
100 g almonds, finely ground
1 teaspoon vanilla essence
2 tablespoons apple juice concentrate

- Preheat the oven to 200°C. Lightly grease a 21 cm pie dish.

- Roll out half the pastry to fit the base and sides of the dish and bake blind according to the instructions on page 107. Allow the base to cool before filling.

- To make the Filling, place the first four ingredients plus a cup of water in a small saucepan and bring to the boil.

- Add the remaining ¼ cup water to the cornflour, stir to make a paste, then add to the lemon mixture, stirring continuously as it boils and thickens. Cook for 2 minutes, remove from heat and cool slightly before pouring into the base.

- Allow the lemon filling to cool and firm up before adding the meringue topping.

- Preheat the oven to 200°C.

- To make the Meringue, beat the egg whites until stiff. Add the other ingredients, one at a time, mixing well after each addition. Spoon the mixture over the lemon filling.

- Bake for 10–15 minutes or until the top is lightly browned.

MARMALADE & APRICOT BREAD PUDDING

8 fresh apricots

8 slices white high-fibre bread, crusts on

¼ cup sugar-free marmalade

2 cups low-fat milk

¼ cup cornflour

2 tablespoons apple juice concentrate

2 eggs or 3 egg whites

1 tablespoon vanilla essence

icing sugar for dusting

- Place the apricots in a saucepan, cover with water and gently poach until the apricots are soft. Drain, halve and remove the stones.

- Preheat the oven to 170°C. Lightly grease a rectangular baking dish.

- Spread the slices of bread with marmalade and cut each piece in half.

- Place a layer of bread on the base of the baking dish and top with apricots.

- Beat together all the remaining ingredients except the icing sugar and pour over the apricots.

- Top with another layer of bread and press down.

- Bake for 30–40 minutes or until the pudding is golden brown. Dust lightly with icing sugar and serve with yoghurt.

RASPBERRY & BANANA PUDDINGS WITH PASSIONFRUIT SAUCE

Serves
6–12

1½ cups unbleached self-raising flour

½ cup unbleached plain flour

1 teaspoon cinnamon

1 cup raspberries, fresh or frozen

2 bananas, peeled and diced

½ cup grapeseed oil

½ cup apple juice concentrate

¾ cup low-fat milk or soymilk

2 eggs or 3 egg whites

icing sugar for dusting

1 quantity Passionfruit Sauce (see
     page 103)

- Preheat the oven to 180°C. Lightly grease a 6- or 12-capacity muffin tray.

- Sift the flours and cinnamon into a bowl. Fold in the raspberries and bananas.

- Combine the grapeseed oil, apple juice concentrate, milk and eggs or egg whites. Beat together and fold into the flour and fruit mixture.

- Spoon the mixture evenly into the prepared tray and bake for 20–30 minutes or until the puddings are golden brown on top.

- Remove from the muffin tray and place on a serving plate. Dust lightly with icing sugar and spoon over some passionfruit sauce.

RASPBERRY & CURRANT BREAD PUDDING

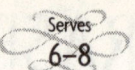

Serves
6–8

You can change the flavours of this pudding by macerating the currants
in just a little brandy, rum or your favourite liqueur.

8 slices wholemeal or grain bread,   2 teaspoons vanilla essence
    crusts on   ¼ cup cornflour
⅓ cup sugar-free raspberry jam   1–2 tablespoons apple juice
1 cup currants   concentrate
2 cups low-fat milk   icing sugar for dusting
2 eggs or 3 egg whites

- Preheat the oven to 170°C. Lightly grease a rectangular
  baking dish.

- Spread the slices of bread with raspberry jam and cut
  each piece in half.

- Place a layer of bread on the base of the baking dish and
  top with currants.

- Beat together all the remaining ingredients except the
  icing sugar and pour over the currants. Top with another
  layer of bread and press down.

- Bake for 30–40 minutes or until the pudding is golden
  brown and crisp on top. Dust lightly with icing sugar and
  serve with Basic Custard (see page 99) or ice-cream.

RICE & SULTANA PUDDING

Serves 6–8

An old-fashioned dessert that is quick, easy and economical to make. It is best to use short-grain rice for rice puddings because the starch tends to break down quickly and acts as a thickening agent. If you have leftover rice you can bypass the first cooking step by adding the cooked rice to the milk, gently heating it and then following the other steps. You can also use honey or maple syrup in place of the apple juice concentrate, but halve the quantities as they contain more sugar.

200 g Arborio short-grain rice

3 cups low-fat milk

1 stick cinnamon

¼ cup apple juice concentrate

2 eggs or 3 egg whites

1 tablespoon vanilla essence

½ cup sultanas or raisins

1 tablespoon finely grated orange zest

icing sugar for dusting

- Place the rice, 2 cups milk and cinnamon in a heavy-based saucepan, stir thoroughly, cover and very slowly heat the milk and rice. The milk should not boil, but only gently simmer for about 15 minutes. Remove from the heat. Stir once or twice during the cooking time and allow the rice to stand until it is soft. Remove the cinnamon stick.

- Beat together the remaining milk, apple juice concentrate, eggs or egg whites and vanilla essence.

- Fold in the sultanas and orange zest. Add this mixture to the rice. >

- Preheat the oven to 180°C. Lightly grease a shallow
  baking dish and pour in the rice mixture.

- Place the baking dish in a tray of warm water that
  comes halfway up the sides of the dish and bake for
  35–40 minutes.

- Dust lightly with icing sugar and serve warm or cold.

TARTS, FLANS & GALETTES

Tarts, flans and galettes provide yet another delightful way to serve fruit as a dessert or as a more substantial afternoon tea treat, or perhaps even for a late Sunday brunch. Crisp light pastry bases, crusty pizza-like bases or wholemeal rich pastry cases hold or enclose decoratively arranged fruits or custard and fruit combinations.

These desserts are ideal served warm or cold. Cut into a triangular wedge, dust lightly with icing sugar or serve with custard, yoghurt or low-fat ricotta cream.

APPLE & APRICOT GALETTE

Serves
6–8

A simple and elegant dessert.

1 quantity Galette Pastry (see   thinly sliced
  page 106)   2 tablespoons lemon juice
¾ cup sugar-free apricot jam   cinnamon
4 Granny Smith apples, cored and

- Preheat the oven to 200°C.

- Roll out the pastry to a 23 cm round and place on a non-stick or lightly greased baking tray. Turn the pastry edges back on themselves so they are slightly raised.

- Spread the pastry with ½ cup of the apricot jam.

- Add the sliced apple in a decorative overlapping pattern.

- Combine the remaining apricot jam with lemon juice and brush over the top of the apple.

- Sprinkle liberally with cinnamon and bake for 15–20 minutes.

- Serve hot with yoghurt or Citrus Custard (see page 101).

APPLE & DATE TART

Serves
8–10

1 quantity Cinnamon Pastry (see
   page 106) or 1 quantity Wholemeal
   Hazelnut Pastry (see page 108)
1 tablespoon apple juice concentrate
1 tablespoon water

FILLING
6 Granny Smith apples, peeled, cored
   and thinly sliced
250 g dates, stoned and chopped
1 cup freshly squeezed orange juice
2 tablespoons lemon juice
1 tablespoon finely grated lemon zest

- To make the Filling, combine all the ingredients in a
  saucepan, cover and gently poach until the apples and
  dates are soft and all liquid is absorbed, about
  15–20 minutes. Allow the mixture to cool.

- Preheat the oven to 220°C. Lightly grease a shallow
  23 cm round fluted flan dish.

- Roll out ⅔ of the pastry on a lightly floured bench to fit
  the base and sides of the prepared dish.

- Transfer the pastry to the dish, being careful not to
  stretch the pastry or it will shrink back during cooking.
  Prick the base with a fork, trim the edges and refrigerate
  for 30 minutes. Place the remaining pastry in a plastic bag
  and refrigerate.

- Spoon the filling over the pastry base. Roll out the
  remaining pastry on a lightly floured bench to form a
  23 cm circle and transfer to the top of the tart. Press the
  edges together to seal and trim away any excess. >

- Cut small vents into the pastry so that steam can escape during cooking.

- Combine the apple juice concentrate and water and use to brush the edges and top of the tart.

- Bake for 40 minutes or until the pastry is golden brown. Serve warm or cold.

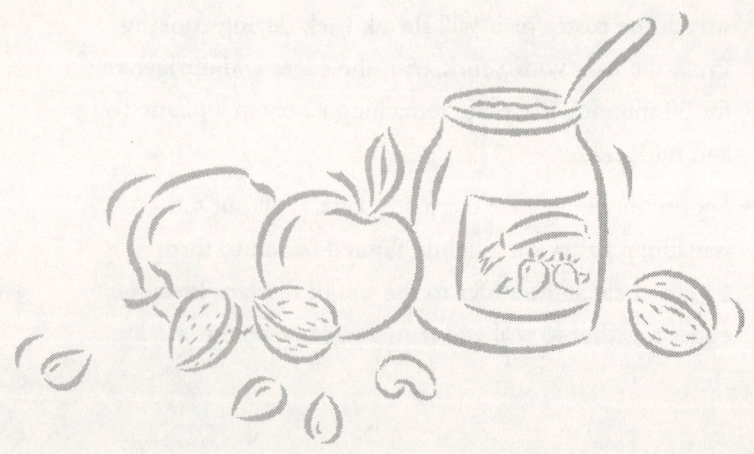

APPLE CUSTARD FLAN

Serves
8–10

BASE

6–8 sheets filo pastry

2 tablespoons apple juice concentrate

2 tablespoons water

FILLING

3 red-skinned apples, cored

¼ cup lemon juice

¼ cup apple juice concentrate

½ cup freshly squeezed orange juice

½ teaspoon cinnamon

¼ teaspoon agar powder

2 cups Basic Custard (see page 99)

icing sugar for dusting

- Preheat the oven to 200°C. Lightly grease a 23 cm round fluted flan dish.

- To make the Base, place the filo pastry on a slightly damp tea towel and cover with another tea towel or plastic wrap so that the pastry does not dry out while you are working.

- Combine the apple juice concentrate and water.

- Place a sheet of filo on the baking paper and brush with a little of the diluted apple juice. Place another sheet of pastry on top and repeat until all the pastry is used up.

- Carefully lift the pastry and mould it to fit the flan dish to create an interesting, rustic-looking pastry case with edges as high as you can make them. Brush the case with the diluted apple juice and bake for 10–12 minutes or until crisp and golden brown. Remove the pastry case from the flan dish immediately and place on a wire cooling tray so that it does not become moist. >

- To make the Filling, slice each apple into 16 thin wedges, place in a shallow pan, pour over the lemon juice, apple juice concentrate, orange juice and cinnamon, cover and simmer until the apple slices are just tender. Carefully remove the apples and set aside.

- Add the agar powder to the pan, stir and simmer until the agar has dissolved and the glaze reduced by about a third.

- Pour the cooled custard into the base of the pastry case. Place the apple slices over the custard in an overlapping circular pattern and spoon over the glaze.

- Allow the pie to cool before serving. Dust the edges of pastry lightly with icing sugar just before serving.

APPLE & SULTANA FLAN

Serves 8–10

1 quantity Sweet Pastry (see page 107)
   or ½ quantity Wholemeal Hazelnut
   Pastry (see page 108)

FILLING

1 kg Granny Smith apples, peeled,
   cored and sliced or
   1 × 825 g can unsweetened
   pie apples

1 cup sultanas

2 tablespoons lemon juice

1 tablespoon Amaretto liqueur

1 cup unsweetened apple juice

1 tablespoon apple juice concentrate

1 teaspoon agar powder

2 Granny Smith apples, cored

- Preheat the oven to 180°C. Have ready a shallow 23 cm round fluted flan dish.

- Prepare and blind bake a pastry case as described on page 107. Allow the case to cool on a wire rack before filling.

- To make the Filling, cover the fresh apples with water and cook until just tender. Drain well and purée. If using canned pie apples, purée.

- Soak the sultanas in lemon juice and liqueur until the sultanas are plump. If you are in a hurry, place them in a microwave for about a minute to achieve the same result.

- Add the sultanas and juices to the puréed apple and mix well. Spoon into the base of the cooked pastry case.

- Combine the apple juice, apple juice concentrate and agar powder in a saucepan and gently simmer until the agar is dissolved. >

- Slice the rest of the apples very thinly and add to the hot
  agar mixture. Allow the apples to become just slightly
  tender and coated with the agar mixture before placing
  them decoratively in a circular pattern over the top of
  the puréed apple. Spoon the glaze over the top of flan.

- Refrigerate the flan so that it firms up before slicing
  and serving.

APRICOT & ALMOND TART

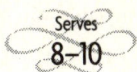

Serves
8–10

1 quantity Cinnamon Pastry (see
  page 106) or 1 quantity Wholemeal
  Pecan Pastry (see page 108)
1 tablespoon apple juice concentrate
1 tablespoon water
¼ cup flaked almonds
icing sugar for dusting

FILLING
2 × 425 g cans unsweetened pie
  apricots
1 tablespoon finely grated orange zest

- Preheat the oven to 200°C. Lightly grease a shallow
  23 cm round fluted flan dish.

- Roll out ⅔ of the pastry on a lightly floured bench to fit
  the base and sides of the dish.

- Transfer the pastry to the dish, being careful not to
  stretch the pastry or it will shrink back during cooking.
  Prick the base with a fork, trim the edges and refrigerate
  for 30 minutes. Place the remaining pastry in a plastic bag
  and refrigerate.

- To make the Filling, combine the apricots and the
  orange zest.

- Spoon the filling over the pastry base. Roll out the
  remaining pastry on a lightly floured bench to form a
  23 cm circle and transfer to the top of the tart. Press the
  edges together to seal and trim away any excess.

- Cut small vents into the pastry so that steam can escape
  during cooking. >

- Combine the apple juice concentrate and water and use
  to brush the edges and top of the tart.

- Scatter almonds over the top and bake for 40–45
  minutes or until the pastry and almonds are
  golden brown.

- Dust lightly with icing sugar and serve with ice-cream or
  Citrus Custard (see page 101).

BLUEBERRY FLAN

Serves
8–10

*You can very successfully turn this into a mulberry or blackberry flan,
or try a combination of all three berries.*

1 quantity Sweet Pastry (see page 107)
  or ½ quantity Wholemeal Almond
  Pastry (see page 108)

FILLING
800 g blueberries, fresh or frozen

2 cups unsweetened apple juice or
  water
½ cup apple juice concentrate
2 tablespoons lemon juice
3 teaspoons agar powder

- Preheat the oven to 180°C. Have ready a shallow 23 cm round fluted flan dish.

- Prepare and blind bake a pastry case as described on page 107. Allow the case to cool on a wire rack before filling.

- To make the Filling, reserve 100 g berries, place all the other ingredients in a saucepan and gently simmer until the agar is dissolved. Remove from the heat.

- Return the reserved berries to the mixture, stir gently so as not to break the berries and allow the mixture to cool slightly before pouring into the pastry case.

- Allow the flan to cool on the bench before refrigerating. Serve with ice-cream or yoghurt.

BRANDY STRAWBERRY FLAN

Serves
8

BASE

6–8 sheets filo pastry

2 tablespoons apple juice concentrate

2 tablespoons water

FILLING

3 cups Basic Custard (see page 99)

500 g strawberries, hulled and halved

GLAZE

2 cups unsweetened apple juice

¼ cup apple juice concentrate

½ cup sugar-free strawberry jam

3 teaspoons agar powder

2 tablespoons brandy

- Preheat the oven to 200°C. Lightly grease a round 23 cm fluted flan dish.

- To make the Base, place the filo pastry on a slightly damp tea towel and cover with another tea towel or plastic wrap so that the pastry does not dry out while you are working.

- Combine the apple juice concentrate and water.

- Place a sheet of filo on the baking paper and brush with a little of the diluted apple juice concentrate. Place another sheet of pastry on top and repeat until all the pastry is used up.

- Carefully lift the pastry and mould it to fit the flan dish to create an interesting, rustic-looking pastry case with edges as high as you can make them. Brush the case with the diluted apple juice and bake for 10–12 minutes or until crisp and golden brown.

- Remove the pastry case from the flan dish immediately and place on a wire cooling tray so that it does not become moist.

- Pour the custard into the pastry case. Top with strawberries.

- To make the Glaze, place all the ingredients in a aucepan, gently simmer, stirring, until the agar has dissolved and the glaze has reduced by half. Allow the glaze to cool slightly before spooning over the strawberries.

- Refrigerate until firm.

FRESH FRUIT CUSTARD TARTLETS

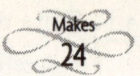

Makes
24

BASE	FILLING
6–8 sheets filo pastry	2 cups Basic Custard (see page 99)
3 tablespoons apple juice concentrate	fresh fruit such as kiwifruit, nectarines,
3 tablespoons water	mangoes, berries, bananas, grapes,
	passionfruit, apricot, peaches

- Preheat the oven to 200°C. Lightly grease a patty tray.

- Place the filo pastry on a slightly damp tea towel and cover with another tea towel or plastic wrap so that the pastry does not dry out while you are working.

- Combine the apple juice concentrate and water. Then place a sheet of filo on the baking paper and brush with some diluted apple juice concentrate. Place another sheet of pastry on top and repeat until all the pastry is used up.

- Using a sharp 6.5 round scone cutter, cut out small rounds of pastry and place on the prepared patty tray.

- Place a few dried beans on a square of baking paper in each pastry round to stop it lifting while cooking.

- Bake for 10 minutes or until the pastry is crisp and golden brown. Remove the beans and allow to cool on a wire cooling rack.

- Place a small spoonful of custard into each pastry round and top with slices of your favourite fruits.

- These tartlets can also be glazed with Cake and Flan Glaze (see page 109).

FRUIT MINCE FLAN

Serves
6-8

*This is one of those recipes that takes only minutes if you have the
fruit mince already made up. I like to make a large batch of fruit mince
in preparation for Christmas; many treats can then be made at a drop
of a hat should unexpected visitors call in.*

1 quantity Sweet Pastry (see page 107)   TOPPING
  or ½ quantity Wholemeal Almond   200 g ricotta
  Pastry (see page 108)   200 g low-fat sour cream or low-fat
4 cups Fruit Mince (see page 109)   yoghurt
                                         ½ teaspoon grated nutmeg

- Preheat the oven to 180°C. Have ready a shallow
  23 cm round fluted flan dish.

- Prepare and blind bake a pastry case as described on
  page 107. Allow the case to cool on a wire rack before
  filling.

- Spread fruit mince evenly over the pastry case.

- To make the Topping, beat together all the ingredients
  except for the nutmeg until smooth.

- Spread the topping evenly over the top of the fruit
  mince.

- Sprinkle nutmeg over the top of flan. Chill before
  serving.

LEMON CUSTARD FLAN

Serves
8–10

1 quantity Sweet Pastry (see page 107)

FILLING

2 cups Basic Custard (see page 99)

1 quantity Lemon Sauce (see page 101)

- Preheat the oven to 180°C. Have ready a shallow 23 cm round fluted flan dish.

- Prepare and blind bake a pastry case as described on page 107. Allow the case to cool on a wire rack before filling.

- Pour the cooled custard into the pastry case and allow it to become firm before pouring over the cooled lemon sauce.

- Refrigerate until the lemon mixture has set.

MANGO &
PASSIONFRUIT
CITRUS FLAN

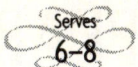

Serves
6–8

BASE

200 g dried apricots

200 g dried apples

1 cup almonds

½ cup coconut

1½ cups rolled oats

2 teaspoons finely grated orange zest

2 tablespoons apple juice concentrate

2 tablespoons freshly squeezed orange
    juice

FILLING

1 litre Basic Custard (see page 99)

2 mangoes, peeled and thinly sliced

¼ cup passionfruit pulp

1 cup Cake and Flan Glaze (see page 109)

- To make the Base, place the apricots, apples, almonds, coconut, rolled oats and orange zest in a food processor and blend until the mixture resembles fine breadcrumbs.

- With the motor running, pour in the combined apple juice concentrate and orange juice, and continue processing until the mixture begins to stick together. Be careful not to over-process or the mixture will be too sticky.

- Press the mixture into a deep 23 cm round ceramic flan dish. Use a straight-sided glass to even out the sides.

- Pour the slightly cooled custard into the pastry base.

- Top with the mango slices decoratively placed in a circular pattern over the top of the custard and spoon over the passionfruit. Refrigerate for 1 hour.

- Spoon the glaze over the top of the flan. As the glaze sets it will hold the mango and passionfruit in place as well as provide an attractive glossy finish.

PEAR, MARMALADE & PECAN GALETTE

1 quantity Galette Pastry (see page 106)

½ cup sugar-free marmalade

6 pears, cored and thinly sliced

2 tablespoons water

2 tablespoons finely chopped pecans

- Preheat the oven to 200°C.

- Roll out the pastry to a 23 cm round and place on a baking tray.

- Turn the pastry edges back on themselves so that they are slightly raised.

- Spread the pastry with the marmalade, reserving a tablespoon of jam.

- Add the sliced pears in a decorative circular overlapping pattern.

- Combine the remaining marmalade with water and rush the tops of the pears.

- Sprinkle with pecans and bake for 15–20 minutes.

- Serve hot with yoghurt or Citrus Custard (see page 101).

PINEAPPLE FRUIT MINCE FLAN

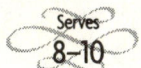

Serves
8–10

1 quantity Sweet Pastry (see page 107)

FILLING

*1 × 400 g can unsweetened crushed
  pineapple*

600 g Fruit Mince (see page 109)

¼ cup cornflour

- Preheat the oven to 180°C. Have ready a shallow 23 cm round fluted flan dish.

- Prepare and blind bake a pastry case as described on page 107. Allow the case to cool on a wire rack before filling.

- To make the Filling, drain the pineapple, reserving the juices. Add the pineapple to the fruit mince.

- Add enough water to the reserved pineapple juice to make up 2 cups of liquid. Mix some of the liquid with the cornflour to make a paste.

- Place the fruit mince, pineapple mixture and pineapple juice in a saucepan and gently simmer. Stir in the cornflour mixture and keep stirring until the mixture boils and thickens.

- Allow the mixture to cool slightly in the saucepan before spooning into the pastry case. Refrigerate until firm. Serve with Citrus Custard (see page 101), ice-cream or yoghurt.

STRANBERRY CUSTARD TARTS

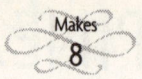

Makes
8

1 quantity Sweet Pastry (see page 107)   400 g strawberries, hulled and thinly
                                           sliced

FILLING   1 quantity Cake and Flan Glaze (see
2 cups Basic Custard (see page 99)   page 109)

- Preheat the oven to 180°C. Lightly grease 8 × 8 cm
  round fluted pie dishes.

- Prepare the pastry as described on page 107, knead
  on a lightly floured bench and cut into 8 equal portions.
  Roll out each portion to fit the base and sides of the
  prepared dishes.

- Transfer each pastry round to the individual pie dishes,
  being careful not to stretch the pastry or it will shrink
  back when you cook it. Prick the bases with a fork, trim
  the edges and refrigerate for 30 minutes.

- Bake the cases for 10 minutes, or until crisp and brown.

- Cool on a wire rack before filling with custard. Top with
  sliced strawberries and brush with hot glaze.

SAUCES & CUSTARDS

Sweet and tangy, delicious fruit sauces can be made simply by thickening some fresh fruit juice, fruit purées or sugar-free jams with a little cornflour. They can be served hot or cold over cakes, pies, puddings and ice-creams. You can add the zest of oranges, lemons, mandarins and grapefruit for sweet and sour flavour variations.

Low-fat custards can be made by combining low-fat milk or soymilk with a thickening agent like cornflour, and they can be sweetened with a sugar substitute such as apple juice concentrate. Finely grated orange zest gives a lovely orange colour as well as a delicate citrusy flavour.

All sauces should be kept refrigerated.

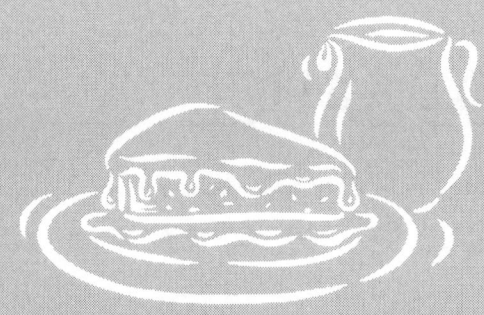

APPLE SAUCE

Serves
6–8

This sauce can be served warm or cold. Add a little apple juice concentrate or cook the apples in fresh orange juice for a sweeter sauce.

6 Granny Smith apples, peeled, cored
   and sliced
half a lemon
1 teaspoon cinnamon

1 cup water
1 tablespoon cornflour
1 tablespoon water, extra

- Place the apples, lemon, cinnamon and water in a saucepan, cover and cook over a slow heat until the apples soften.

- Remove the lemon and purée the apples. For a chunkier apple sauce, purée only half the mixture and combine the two.

- Mix the water and cornflour to make a paste, stir through the cooked apple mixture and continue cooking until the sauce boils and thickens. Add the extra tablespoon of water if you feel the sauce is too thick.

APRICOT SAUCE

1 cup sugar-free apricot jam
1 cup water

1 tablespoon Amaretto liqueur
1 teaspoon grated orange zest

- Place all the ingredients in a saucepan and keep stirring until the jam breaks down and thickens.

- The longer you cook the sauce, the richer the flavour and the thicker its consistency.

BASIC CUSTARD

Serves
4-6

*This recipe is ideal for desserts that require a custard to set firm. It can
be made with low-fat milk or soymilk. The orange zest colours the
custard as well as adding flavour. The yoghurt adds a creamy texture.*

INGREDIENT	MAKES	MAKES	MAKES	MAKES
MILK	2 cups	3 cups	1 litre	2 litres
CORNFLOUR	½ cup	¾ cup	1 cup	2 cups
VANILLA ESSENCE	1 tspn	1½ tspn	2 tspn	1 tbsp
ORANGE ZEST	2 tspn	1 tbsp	1 tbsp	2 tbsp
APPLE JUICE CONCENTRATE	¼ cup	⅓ cup	½ cup	1 cup
LOW-FAT YOGHURT	½ cup	¾ cup	1 cup	2 cups

- Mix a little milk with the cornflour to make a paste.

- Add the cornflour mixture to the remaining milk,
  vanilla and orange zest in a saucepan and slowly bring to
  the boil, stirring continuously until the custard begins
  to thicken.

- Remove the custard from the heat and stir in the apple
  juice concentrate and yoghurt.

BLUEBERRY SAUCE

Serves
4–6

For a chunkier blueberry sauce, reserve a cup of blueberries and gently stir into the sauce once it has boiled and thickened. For a change in flavour try adding a pinch of cinnamon or nutmeg or a few cloves.

2 cups unsweetened pear juice or water

¼ cup cornflour

⅓ cup apple juice concentrate

450 g blueberries, fresh or frozen

1 tablespoon lemon juice

- Mix a little pear juice or water with the cornflour to make a paste.
- Place the remaining pear juice or water, cornflour mixture and all the other ingredients in a saucepan and slowly bring to the boil, stirring continuously until the sauce boils and thickens.

CHOCOLATE SAUCE

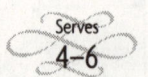
Serves
4–6

This sauce can be served with hot puddings, over pancakes or with a favourite ice-cream. It is also delicious with fresh berries.

1 tablespoon cocoa or 2–3 teaspoons carob powder

2 tablespoons cornflour

1 cup low-fat milk or soymilk

2 tablespoons apple juice concentrate

1 teaspoon vanilla essence

- Mix the cocoa or carob and cornflour with a little milk to make a paste.
- Add this to the remaining milk, apple juice concentrate and vanilla essence in a saucepan and slowly bring to the boil. Keep stirring until the sauce boils and thickens.

CITRUS CUSTARD

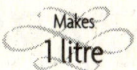

Makes
1 litre

3 cups low-fat milk or soymilk

½ cup cornflour

1 tablespoon grated orange zest

1 teaspoon finely grated lemon or
   lime zest

¼ cup apple juice concentrate

½ cup freshly squeezed orange juice

- Mix some milk with the cornflour to make a paste.

- Place the remaining milk, orange zest, lemon or lime zest, apple juice concentrate and cornflour mixture in a saucepan. Slowly simmer until the custard begins to boil and thicken.

- Remove the custard from the heat and stir in the orange juice (add more or less orange juice for a thinner or thicker consistency).

LEMON SAUCE

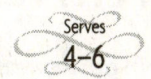

Serves
4–6

This tangy sauce complements fresh fruits, is perfect with pancakes and makes an excellent tart and cake filling. For a thinner pouring consistency, reduce the amount of cornflour.

1¼ cups water

¼ cup cornflour

¾ cup freshly squeezed lemon juice

½ cup apple juice concentrate

½ teaspoon orange essence

grated zest of an orange

- Mix some water with the cornflour to make a paste.

- Place the remaining water, cornflour mixture and all the other ingredients in a saucepan and slowly bring to the boil. Keep stirring until the mixture boils and thickens.

MARSALA CUSTARD

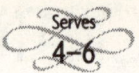

Serves
4–6

3 cups low-fat milk or soymilk

¼ cup cornflour

1 tablespoon grated orange zest

2 tablespoons apple juice concentrate

2 tablespoons marsala

2 tablespoons freshly squeezed
  orange juice

1 tablespoon marsala, extra

- Mix some milk with the cornflour to make a paste.

- Place the remaining milk, orange zest, apple juice
  concentrate, marsala and cornflour mixture in a saucepan.
  Simmer until the custard begins to boil and thicken.

- Remove the custard from the heat and stir in the orange
  juice (add more or less orange juice for a thinner or
  thicker consistency) and marsala.

MIXED BERRY SAUCE

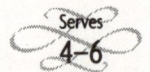

Serves
4–6

1½ cups unsweetened apple or
  pear juice

¼ cup cornflour

500 g mixed seasonal berries, stems
  removed

⅓ cup apple juice concentrate

1 tablespoon lemon juice

- Mix a little apple or pear juice with the cornflour to
  make a paste.

- Set aside a cup of the fruit.

- Add all the ingredients and the cornflour mixture to a
  saucepan and slowly bring to the boil, stirring
  continuously, but gently, so as not to break up the fruit.

- Remove the sauce from the heat and gently stir in the
  remaining berries.

ORANGE CITRUS SAUCE

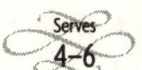
Serves 4-6

This sauce is simple to make and is especially good after a hot curry dish. Try it over cakes as a glaze, and with tarts and puddings in place of cream or ice-cream.

2 cups freshly squeezed orange juice

2 tablespoons cornflour

grated zest of an orange

grated zest of a lemon or lime

½ cup apple juice concentrate

- Mix some orange juice with cornflour to make a paste.
- Place the remaining ingredients and cornflour mixture in a saucepan and slowly bring to the boil, stirring continuously until the sauce boils and thickens.

PASSIONFRUIT SAUCE

Serves 4-6

2 cups freshly squeezed orange juice

¼ cup cornflour

1 cup passionfruit pulp

1–2 tablespoons brandy or orange-flavoured liqueur

- Mix some orange juice with cornflour to make a paste.
- Place the remaining ingredients and cornflour mixture in a saucepan and slowly bring to the boil, stirring continuously until the sauce boils and thickens.
- This sauce can be served hot or cold. You can strain the seeds from the passionfruit juice if you desire.

RASPBERRY & PEACH SAUCE

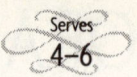
Serves
4–6

If you want this sauce to be a little sweeter, add some apple juice concentrate. Serve it over fresh fruits or drizzle it over a firm yoghurt.

500 g raspberries

4 yellow clingstone peaches, peeled
 and stoned

2 teaspoons Galliano liqueur

apple juice concentrate

- Combine all the ingredients except the apple juice concentrate in a blender and purée until smooth.

- Taste. If it is sweet enough, do not add any apple juice concentrate or add just a little at a time until the sauce is sweet enough to your liking.

RASPBERRY SAUCE

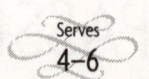
Serves
4–6

This sauce tastes as good cold as it does warm and is particularly good with pancakes. It is delicious served over hot apple strudel and fabulous simply served with a big bowl of strawberries.

½ cup water

1 tablespoon cornflour

1 teaspoon lemon juice

¼ cup apple juice concentrate

600 g raspberries, fresh or frozen

- Mix the water and cornflour to make a paste.

- Place the remaining ingredients and cornflour mixture in a saucepan and slowly bring to the boil, stirring continuously until the sauce boils and thickens.

PASTRY & OTHER BASIC RECIPES

*P*astry is traditionally very high in fat. The pastry recipes here are excellent low-fat alternatives that fulfil the purpose of pastry – to hold or enclose a filling besides adding a complementary flavour or texture to the filling used.

CINNAMON PASTRY

Makes enough to line the base, sides and top of a 23 cm dish.

2 cups unbleached plain flour	1/3 cup grapeseed oil
2 tablespoons icing sugar	2/3 cup cold water
2 teaspoons cinnamon	

- Combine the flour, icing sugar and cinnamon in a bowl.

- Stir in the grapeseed oil and enough water to make a soft dough. Form the dough into a ball, wrap in plastic and refrigerate for 30 minutes.

- Roll out according to the recipe or roll out the pastry to fit a baking dish and refrigerate for 30 minutes before cooking. Refer to page 107 for instructions on baking blind.

GALETTE PASTRY

Makes a 25 cm round base.

1 cup unbleached plain flour	1/4 cup grapeseed oil
2 tablespoons icing sugar	2 tablespoons cold water

- Combine the flour and icing sugar in a bowl.

- Stir in the grapeseed oil and enough water to make a soft dough. Form the dough into a ball, wrap in plastic and refrigerate for 30 minutes.

- Roll out according to the recipe.

SWEET PASTRY

Makes enough to line the base and sides of a 23 cm pie dish or 8 × 8 cm pie dishes.

1 cup unbleached plain flour

1 cup rolled oats

⅓ cup grapeseed oil

2 tablespoons apple juice concentrate

¼ cup cold water

- Combine the flour and rolled oats in a bowl.

- Stir in the grapeseed oil and apple juice concentrate and enough water to make a soft dough. Form the dough into a ball, wrap in plastic and refrigerate for 30 minutes.

- Roll out according to the recipe or roll out the pastry to fit a baking dish and refrigerate for 30 minutes before cooking.

- Baking the pastry blind will give you the best results.

- To bake blind, preheat the oven to 180–200°C. Cut out a circle of baking paper to fit the base of the tin. Roll out the pastry and line the tin. Cover the base with the paper and sprinkle over some brown rice or dried beans to act as a weight during the first stage of cooking.

- Bake for 8–10 minutes, remove the weights and paper, and bake for another 5 minutes to allow the base to brown evenly. Cool before using.

WHOLEMEAL PECAN PASTRY

Makes enough to line the base, sides and top of a 23 cm pie dish or the base, sides and lattice top.

1 cup unbleached wholemeal self-
  raising flour
¾ cup unbleached plain flour

50 g finely ground pecans
⅓ cup grapeseed oil
½ cup cold water

- Combine the flours and ground pecans in a bowl.

- Stir in the grapeseed oil and enough water to make a soft dough. Form the dough into a ball, wrap in plastic and refrigerate for 30 minutes.

- Roll out according to the recipe. Refer to page 107 for instructions on baking blind.

- To make WHOLEMEAL ALMOND PASTRY, substitute ground almonds for pecans.

- To make WHOLEMEAL HAZELNUT PASTRY, substitute ground hazelnuts for pecans.

CAKE & FLAN GLAZE

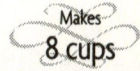

Makes 1 cup

1 cup water, unsweetened apple, pear
  or orange juice

1 tablespoon apple juice concentrate

1 teaspoon agar powder

- Combine all the ingredients in a saucepan. Simmer, stirring continuously, until the glaze boils and agar is thoroughly dissolved. Cool slightly before using.

FRUIT MINCE

Makes 8 cups

250 g currants

250 g sultanas

250 g raisins

250 g mixed peel

1½ teaspoons cinnamon

1 teaspoon mixed spice

1 teaspoon nutmeg

2 tablespoons brandy

2 tablespoons apple juice concentrate

3 Granny Smith apples, peeled and
  grated

1 tablespoon cornflour

4 cups unsweetened apple juice

- Place all the ingredients except the cornflour and ¼ cup unsweetened apple juice in a saucepan. Cover and bring to the boil. Lower the heat and simmer uncovered for 30 minutes.

- Combine the cornflour and apple juice, and stir through the hot fruit mixture. Continue cooking, stirring continuously for 10 minutes or until the mixture has thickened.

- Allow the mixture to cool. It keeps in the refrigerator for up to 3 months.

RICOTTA CREAM

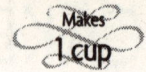

300 g low-fat ricotta   *2–3 teaspoons vanilla essence*

¼ cup low-fat milk

- Purée all the ingredients together until smooth. Keep in
  the refrigerator and use within 2 days.

ABOUT THE INGREDIENTS

AGAR This is a seaweed setting agent like gelatine. It is high in protein and calcium, and easy to digest. One teaspoon of agar powder sets approximately one cup of liquid, depending on the texture you require.

ALMONDS Although almonds have a high fat content, they are a high-quality, nutritious food. However, to reduce fat intake in the diet it is important to keep recipes containing almonds to a minimum. Almonds are best bought in their shells and shelled as required. Unshelled nuts are protected from heat, air, light and moisture and store well.

APPLE JUICE CONCENTRATE A concentrated apple juice used as a substitute for sugar. It is about 66 per cent sugar compared to honey, which is about 80 per cent sugar.

APPLES Apples are available all year round and the many varieties provide a host of tastes and textures. They are low in kilojoules, high in vitamin C and an excellent carbohydrate food. Not only does the pectin in apples add lots of flavour and moisture to recipes, it also provides extra natural fibre. Canned pie apples with no added sugar have the same nutritional value as fresh apples, so for convenience always keep a couple of cans in your pantry. All other fruits and most spices combine well with apple.

BAKING POWDER This fine, white powder, high in sodium but unlike bicarbonate of soda, is an excellent source of calcium and phosphorus. When heated it emits carbon dioxide that causes the mixture to which it has been added to become aerated or light in texture. For sodium-free baking powder combine 2 tablespoons each of cornflour, cream of tartar and potassium bicarbonate (available at chemists). Store this mixture in an airtight container and use about 2 teaspoons for every cup of flour. Many health food stores now sell this product.

BANANAS   Bananas, grown in the world's tropical regions, are a good source of vitamin C, contain moderate amounts of fibre and iron, and are especially high in potassium. Bananas are available all year round and although delicious when raw, the flavour of cooked bananas is quite unique. Like apples, bananas go well with almost all fruits. Different spices or a little orange or lemon zest really enhance their overall flavour. Pecans, walnuts or macadamias also combine well with bananas.

BLUEBERRIES   These plump, small, round, juicy berries, with their sweet–tart taste and purple–blue skin, are a delicious dessert ingredient. A native of North America, blueberries are an excellent source of vitamin C and have moderate amounts of iron and fibre.

CAROB   Carob comes from the long pods of the carob tree. It has no significant nutritional value, but its flavour is similar to chocolate; carob is also caffeine-free. Carob buds usually have high levels of added fat and some added sugar,

so use sparingly if on a low-fat, sugar-free diet.

CINNAMON   An aromatic, fragrant spice that goes well with all fruits and imparts a lovely flavour to baked goods.

COCONUT   Use shredded coconut (see page 116). To toast, stir the coconut in a small pan over low heat until the coconut begins to change colour.

COCONUT MILK   Coconut milk is thinner in consistency than coconut cream and lower in fat. If using powdered coconut milk make sure you follow the mixing instructions for coconut milk, not coconut cream.

COLD PRESSED OIL   When oil is extracted with little or no heat – or use of chemical solvents, as happens with ordinary oils – the vitamin E content is not destroyed. Oil should be bought in brown bottles or tins, kept away from the light and refrigerated. Do not use oil excessively and only in the amounts used in the recipes. Grapeseed oil is ideal for sweet recipes.

CORNFLOUR   Used as a thickening agent.

DATES   The date is considered, along with the fig, to be the oldest known of all cultivated fruits. It is an excellent energy food because of its carbohydrate value and contains fibre, some iron, magnesium, niacin, folate and vitamin B6. If the dates are very hard and dry, soak them overnight in water. For extra flavour macerate them in unsweetened fruit juices, brandy, sherry, port, marsala or rum. Drain off any liquid before using. Dates combine particularly well with apples, bananas, apricots, pears and oranges.

DRIED FRUITS   These include apricots, apples, raisins, sultanas, currants, bananas, peaches, nectarines and pears. Dried fruits contain a high level of natural sugar. Look for sun-dried fruits without additives where possible.

EGGS   Egg yolks contain fat and cholesterol. The egg white protein, when whipped to form stiff peaks, breaks down into short strands and these expand to form elastic-walled cells that trap air. The cells in turn expand when heated. This is what makes egg whites such a valuable rising agent. Yolk protein, on the other hand, binds and thickens. It can be substituted by doubling the egg whites for the number of eggs in a recipe or by adding a small amount of another thickening and binding ingredient like arrowroot, grated or cooked apple or fresh banana. All recipes use 55 g eggs.

EVAPORATED SKIM MILK (CANNED)
Milk with a large percentage of water removed. It contains less than 1 per cent fat, no sugar, has a heavier texture than non-fat milk, and is a good substitute in recipes that call for whole milk, sour cream or cream. In recipes that call for evaporated skim milk you can substitute soymilk.

FIGS   The fig tree originated in western Asia and is one of the oldest known cultivated fruit trees. The fruit is high in carbohydrate, rich in fibre and contains magnesium, calcium and iron. Like dates, figs bring sweetness, richness and extra moisture to your recipes and combine especially well with apples, bananas and peaches. The drying process concentrates the kilojoule value as well as the nutritional value of fruit, so don't over-indulge if you want to keep your weight down.

GLACÉ GINGER   Glacé ginger is cooked ginger that has been dipped in hot water to soften the surface, drained, and dipped in a very strong sugary syrup to give it a smooth, glossy finish. To remove the syrup and most of the sugar but not the taste before cooking, run the glacé fruit under warm water and dry on a paper towel.

GREEN GINGER WINE   A sweet wine infused with ginger.

GROUND GINGER   Lends a sweet and warm quality to baked fruits and pastries. Fresh ginger is not a substitute.

LEMONS   The lemon is thought to have originated in the south of China, India and Burma. It is now successfully cultivated in many warm coastal areas around the world where it is used to flavour both sweet and savoury cooking. Like other citrus fruits the lemon is low in kilojoules and high in vitamin C and fibre. Lemon zest heightens the flavour of recipes that use apple, banana, pear, peach or blueberry. Lemons makes delicious sauces and pie fillings.

LOW-FAT COTTAGE CHEESE   This cheese has the consistency of paste and has a light acidic flavour, though it is fairly bland. It contains a maximum of about 0.4 per cent fat. Combined with ricotta, it makes a good low-fat alternative to cream cheese or cream.

LOW-FAT RICOTTA   This is made from milk curds instead of whey (liquid from milk), which is drained off. It has a bland flavour and is a mass of fine, small curd particles. Preferably look for ricotta with 1 per cent fat content.

LOW-FAT SKIM MILK   This is milk with 1 per cent milk fat. It contains the same nutrients of whole milk except for fat-soluble vitamins. It is also available in powdered form that needs to be reconstituted with water before use.

LOW-FAT YOGHURT   A cultivated milk product. Specific bacteria are added to fresh skim milk to develop a tangy flavour, custard-like yoghurt. It is more nutritious than milk because an extra 4 per cent of non-fat milk powder is added to enhance the texture. It has a fat content of approximately 0.1 per cent.

MACADAMIAS   Native to the coastal rainforests of Queensland, Australia, the macadamia is high in oil (mainly unsaturated fat), and is a good source of fibre. The rich, buttery flavour of the nut is enhanced when cooked.

MANGOES   The mango, at its peak in summer, is one of the most delicious tropical fruits. It has a high vitamin A level and lower amounts of iron and vitamin C. Although my favourite way to eat a mango is to peel away the outer skin and devour its fragrant, velvety, smooth flesh, it

also cooks well, especially when combined with other fruits such as bananas and apples. Spices such as cinnamon, ginger and cardamom will complement mango recipes.

PASSIONFRUIT   There are four varieties of passionfruit but the most popular is the purple, which grows best in the subtropical climate. The purple passionfruit is an excellent carbohydrate food with high levels of vitamin C and fibre. Its sharp, sweet flavour is incomparable.

PECANS   The pecan originated in North America and has become a popular addition to many American dishes. It is low in fibre and high in oil, the oil being 95 per cent unsaturated (mainly mono-unsaturated). Pecans impart a wonderfully rich flavour when cooked.

PRUNES   The prune is a dried d'Agen sugar plum. The plum is grown in all corners of the world and traditionally is known for its laxative effect and as an addition to breakfast cereals. Not only is it highly nutritious and high in fibre, vitamin A, iron and phosphorous, but its flavour also enhances fruits like apples, bananas and peaches and vegetables like pumpkins and sweet potatoes. Remove the stone before cooking, and if the prunes have dried out, reconstitute in a little water, fruit juice, port or sherry.

RASPBERRIES   The raspberry was a native of Europe before making its way around the world. It is high in fibre and iron with a significant amount of vitamin C. But its greatest appeal lies in its delicate, sweet, almost wine-like flavour.

RHUBARB   Many people think of rhubarb as a fruit but actually it is a vegetable related to sorrel. Only the pinkish stem of this large perennial plant is used in cooking; the leaves contain dangerous amounts of oxalic acid. Its kilojoule value is low compared to most fruits and it is significantly high in calcium. Walnuts, pecans, cinnamon, mixed spices, cloves, cardamom and ginger complement the flavour of rhubarb.

SHREDDED COCONUT   Coconut is an excellent source of phosphorous and potassium but is high in fat. A small amount is usually called for to flavour a recipe, but use sparingly.

SKIM MILK POWDER   This is milk from which the moisture and fat have been removed. It is either added straight to dry ingredients or reconstituted with water before use.

UNBLEACHED WHITE FLOUR   Similar to white flour, but has not been through the bleaching process. Bleaching (the addition of a chemical called benzoyl peroxide) has no purpose other than to make the flour appear white in colour and is another example of how foods are being chemically interfered with simply to be visually pleasing. Ironically, flour naturally bleaches when stored.

WALNUTS   There are fifteen varieties of walnut, the most popular being the yellow-brown. Walnuts are high in oil and linoleic acid (a polyunsaturated acid). They are also a good source of protein.

Purchase walnuts only as you need them; once shelled they lose their freshness. Store shelled nuts in an air-tight container in the refrigerator.

WHOLEMEAL FLOUR Milled from whole wheat grain with a large proportion of the outer husk remaining in the finished product. It adds texture, a nutty flavour, and essential flavour to your recipes. Wholemeal flour contains more minerals and vitamins than white flour. It is an excellent source of niacin, iron and magnesium, and smaller amounts of protein and zinc.

INDEX

agar 111
almonds 111
   Apple, banana & pineapple strudel 22–3
   Apple oat crumble 25
   Apricot & almond tart 85–6
   Apricot crumble slice 3
   Banana & rhubarb cake 6
   Carob hedgehog balls 9
   Chewy banana & nut slice 12
   Lemon meringue pie 70–1
   Mango & passionfruit citrus flan 93
   Winter fruit salad 36
apple juice concentrate 111
apples 111
   Apple & apricot galette 78
   Apple & date tart 79–80
   Apple & ginger pie 62
   Apple & hazelnut custard cake 2
   Apple & sultana flan 83–4
   Apple, banana & pineapple strudel 22–3
   Apple custard flan 81–2
   Apple dumplings 24
   Apple oat crumble 25
   Apple sauce 98
   Apple strudel 26–7
   Baked apple with fruit filling 29
   Blackberry & apple fruit swirls 54
   Cold Christmas pudding 68
   Festive fruit & nut cake 16–17
   Fruit mince 109
   Watermelon & apple spice sorbet 50
apricots
   Apple & apricot galette 78
   Apricot & almond tart 85–6
   Apricot & passionfruit mousse 52
   Apricot crumble slice 3
   Apricot sauce 98
   Apricot sorbet 39
   Creamy coconut & apricot rice pudding 69
   Fresh fruit custard tartlets 90
   Marmalade & apricot bread pudding 72
Autumn pears 28

Baked apple with fruit filling 29
Baked berry cheesecake with raspberry sauce 4
Baked coconut custard 53
baking powder 111
bananas 112
   Apple, banana & pineapple strudel 22–3
   Banana & rhubarb cake 6
   Banana & ricotta strudel 30–1
   Banana, bourbon & orange cake 5
   Banana fritters 32
   Banana yoghurt pie 63–4

   Chewy banana & nut slice 12
   Chunky banana ice-cream 41
   Fiji cake 18
   Fresh fruit custard tartlets 90
   Raspberry & banana puddings with passionfruit sauce 73
Basic custard 99
berries
   Baked berry cheesecake with raspberry sauce 4
   Berry pudding 65
   Berry streusel cake 7
   Berry summer jelly pudding 66
   Fresh fruit custard tartlets 90
   Mixed berry sauce 102
   Red berry passion fruit salad 35
Blackberry & apple fruit swirls 54
blueberries 112
   Berry streusel cake 7
   Blueberry flan 87
   Blueberry sauce 100
   Blueberry yoghurt fruit swirls 55
Boysenberry ice-cream 40
Brandy strawberry flan 88–9
bread puddings
   Berry pudding 65
   Marmalade & apricot bread pudding 72
   Raspberry & currant bread pudding 74

Cake & flan glaze 109
cakes
   Apple & hazelnut custard cake 2
   Banana & rhubarb cake 6
   Banana, bourbon & orange cake 5
   Berry streusel cake 7
   Carob & date mud cake 8
   Carrot cake with lemon cheese icing 10–11
   Christmas cake 13–14
   Festive fruit & nut cake 16–17
   Fiji cake 18
   Lemon poppyseed ring cake 19
   Pumpkin & prune spice cake 20
carob 112
   Banana yoghurt pie 63–4
   Carob & date mud cake 8
   Carob hedgehog balls 9
   Carob mousse 56
   Chocolate puddings with raspberry sauce 67
   Chocolate sauce 100
   Fiji cake 18
   Rich cream carob & coconut ice-cream 48
Carrot cake with lemon cheese icing 10–11
cheesecakes
   Baked berry cheesecake with raspberry sauce 4
Chewy banana & nut slice 12
Chocolate puddings with raspberry sauce 67

Chocolate sauce 100
Christmas cake 13–14
Chunky banana ice-cream 41
cinnamon 112
    Cinnamon pastry 106
Citrus custard 101
coconut 112, 116
    Apricot crumble slice 3
    Baked coconut custard 53
    Berry streusel cake 7
    Blueberry yoghurt fruit swirls 55
    Carob hedgehog balls 9
    Chewy banana & nut slice 12
    Creamy coconut & apricot rice pudding 69
    Mango & passionfruit citrus flan 93
    Rich cream carob & coconut ice-cream 48
coconut milk 112
Cold Christmas pudding 68
cold pressed oil 112
cornflower 113
cottage cheese, low-fat 114
    Baked berry cheesecake with raspberry sauce 4
    Banana & ricotta strudel 30–1
    Blackberry & apple fruit swirls 54
Creamy coconut & apricot rice pudding 69
crumbles
    Apple oat crumble 25
currants
    Raspberry & currant bread pudding 74
custard
    Apple & hazelnut custard cake 2
    Apple custard flan 81–2
    Baked coconut custard 53
    Basic custard 99
    Citrus custard 101
    Fresh fruit custard tartlets 90
    Lemon custard flan 92
    Marsala custard 102
    Strawberry custard tarts 96

dates 113
    Apple & date tart 79–80
    Banana yoghurt pie 63–4
    Carob & date mud cake 8
    Carob hedgehog balls 9
    Date & pecan torte 15
    Winter fruit salad 36
dried fruits 113
    Baked apple with fruit filling 29
    Carrot cake with lemon cheese icing 10–11
    Chewy banana & nut slice 12
    Christmas cake 13–14
    Cold Christmas pudding 68
    Festive fruit & nut cake 16–17
    Fruit mince 109
    Mango & passionfruit citrus flan 93
    Winter fruit salad 36
dumplings
    Apple dumplings 24

eggs 113
evaporated skim milk (canned) 113

Festive fruit & nut cake 16–17
figs 113–14
Fiji cake 18
flans
    Apple & sultana flan 83–4
    Apple custard flan 81–2
    Blueberry flan 87
    Brandy strawberry flan 88–9
    Cake & flan glaze 109
    Fruit mince flan 91
    Lemon custard flan 92
    Mango & passionfruit citrus flan 93
    Pineapple fruit mince flan 95
Fresh fruit custard tartlets 90
fritters
    Banana fritters 32
Fruit mince 109
    Fruit mince flan 91
    Pineapple fruit mince flan 95
fruit salads
    Jellied fruit salad 57
    Red berry passion fruit salad 35
    Tropical paradise fruit salad 35
    Winter fruit salad 36
fruit swirls
    Blackberry & apple fruit swirls 54
    Blueberry yoghurt fruit swirls 55
    Passionfruit & lemon swirls 58
    Raspberry & walnut fruit swirls 60

galettes
    Apple & apricot galette 78
    Galette pastry 106
    Pear, marmalade & pecan galette 94
ginger
    Apple & ginger pie 62
    Ginger pears 33
    glacé ginger 114
    green ginger wine 114
    ground ginger 114
    Kiwifruit & ginger sorbet 42
glazes
    Cake & flan glaze 109
grapes
    Fresh fruit custard tartlets 90

hazelnuts
    Apple & hazelnut custard cake 2
    Chewy banana & nut slice 12

ice-creams
    Boysenberry ice-cream 40
    Chunky banana ice-cream 41
    Making ice-cream & sorbet 38
    Orange, raisin & macadamia nut ice-cream 43–4
    Passionfruit ice-cream 45

Pineapple & mango ice-cream   47
Rich cream carob & coconut ice-cream   48
Strawberry ice-cream   49
icing
Carrot cake with lemon cheese icing   10–11

jellies
Berry summer jelly pudding   66
Jellied fruit salad   57

kiwifruit
Fresh fruit custard tartlets   90
Jellied fruit salad   57
Kiwifruit & ginger sorbet   42

lemons   114
Carrot cake with lemon cheese icing   10–11
Lemon custard flan   92
Lemon meringue pie   70–1
Lemon mousse   58
Lemon poppyseed ring cake   19
Lemon sauce   101
Passionfruit & lemon swirls   58
Pear & lemon sorbet   46

macadamias   115
Orange, raisin & macadamia nut ice-cream   43–4
mangoes   115
Fiji cake   18
Fresh fruit custard tartlets   90
Jellied fruit salad   57
Mango & passionfruit citrus flan   93
Pineapple & mango ice-cream   47
Tropical paradise fruit salad   35
marmalade
Marmalade & apricot bread pudding   72
Pear, marmalade & pecan galette   94
Marsala custard   102
Mixed berry sauce   102
mousses
Apricot & passionfruit mousse   52
Carob mousse   56
Lemon mousse   58
Peach & yoghurt mousse   59
Raspberry mousse   60

nectarines
Fresh fruit custard tartlets   90
nuts, mixed
Festive fruit & nut cake   16–17

oil, cold pressed   112
oranges
Banana, bourbon & orange cake   5
Jellied fruit salad   57
Orange citrus sauce   103
Orange, raisin & macadamia nut ice-cream   43–4
Tropical paradise fruit salad   35

passionfruit   115
Apricot & passionfruit mousse   52
Fresh fruit custard tartlets   90
Mango & passionfruit citrus flan   93
Passionfruit & lemon swirls   58
Passionfruit ice-cream   45
Passionfruit sauce   103
Raspberry & banana puddings with passionfruit sauce   73
Tropical paradise fruit salad   35
pastry
Cinnamon pastry   106
Galette pastry   106
Sweet pastry   107
Wholemeal pecan pastry   108
pawpaws
Tropical paradise fruit salad   35
peaches
Fresh fruit custard tartlets   90
Jellied fruit salad   57
Peach & yoghurt mousse   59
Poached Amaretto peaches   34
Raspberry & peach sauce   104
pears
Autumn pears   28
Ginger pears   33
Pear & lemon sorbet   46
Pear, marmalade & pecan galette   94
pecans   115
Berry streusel cake   7
Blueberry yoghurt fruit swirls   55
Date & pecan torte   15
Pear, marmalade & pecan galette   94
Wholemeal pecan pastry   108
pies
Apple & ginger pie   62
Banana yoghurt pie   63–4
Lemon meringue pie   70–1
pineapples
Apple, banana & pineapple strudel   22–3
Fiji cake   18
Jellied fruit salad   57
Pineapple & mango ice-cream   47
Pineapple fruit mince flan   95
Pineapple sauce   22–23
Tropical paradise fruit salad   35
Poached Amaretto peaches   34
poppyseeds
Lemon poppyseed ring cake   19
prunes   115–16
Pumpkin & prune spice cake   20
Winter fruit salad   36
puddings
Berry pudding   65
Berry summer jelly pudding   66
Chocolate puddings with raspberry sauce   67
Cold Christmas pudding   68
Creamy coconut & apricot rice pudding   69
Marmalade & apricot bread pudding   72
Raspberry & banana puddings with passionfruit sauce   73

Raspberry & currant bread pudding 74
Rice & sultana pudding 75–6
pumpkin
Christmas cake 13–14
Pumpkin & prune spice cake 20

raisins
Banana & ricotta strudel 30–1
Carob hedgehog balls 9
Orange, raisin & macadamia nut ice-cream 43–4
Rice & sultana pudding 75–6
raspberries 116
Baked berry cheesecake with raspberry sauce 4
Berry streusel cake 7
Chocolate puddings with raspberry sauce 67
Raspberry & banana puddings with passionfruit sauce 73
Raspberry & currant bread pudding 74
Raspberry & peach sauce 104
Raspberry & walnut fruit swirls 60
Raspberry mousse 60
Raspberry sauce 104
Red berry passion fruit salad 35
rhubarb 116
Banana & rhubarb cake 6
rice puddings
Creamy coconut & apricot rice pudding 69
Rice & sultana pudding 75–6
Rich cream carob & coconut ice-cream 48
ricotta, low-fat 114
Baked berry cheesecake with raspberry sauce 4
Banana & ricotta strudel 30–1
Blackberry & apple fruit swirls 54
Fruit mince flan 91
Ricotta cream 110

sauces
Apple sauce 98
Apricot sauce 98
Baked berry cheesecake with raspberry sauce 4
Blueberry sauce 100
Chocolate puddings with raspberry sauce 67
Chocolate sauce 100
Lemon sauce 101
Mixed berry sauce 102
Orange citrus sauce 103
Passionfruit sauce 103
Pineapple sauce 22–23
Raspberry & banana puddings with passionfruit sauce 73
Raspberry & peach sauce 104
Raspberry sauce 104
shredded coconut 116
skim milk

low-fat 114–15
powder 116
slices
Apricot crumble slice 3
Chewy banana & nut slice 12
sorbets
Apricot sorbet 39
Kiwifruit & ginger sorbet 42
Making ice-cream & sorbet 38
Pear & lemon sorbet 46
Watermelon & apple spice sorbet 50
strawberries
Brandy strawberry flan 88–9
Date & pecan torte 15
Jellied fruit salad 57
Strawberry custard tarts 96
Strawberry ice-cream 49
strudels
Apple, banana & pineapple strudel 22–3
Apple strudel 26–7
Banana & ricotta strudel 30–1
sultanas
Apple & sultana flan 83–4
Rice & sultana pudding 75–6
Sweet pastry 107

tarts
Apple & date tart 79–80
Apricot & almond tart 85–6
Fresh fruit custard tartlets 90
Strawberry custard tarts 96
tortes
Date & pecan torte 15
Tropical paradise fruit salad 35

unbleached white flour 116

walnuts 116–17
Banana & ricotta strudel 30–1
Banana fritters 32
Raspberry & walnut fruit swirls 60
watermelons
Red berry passion fruit salad 35
Watermelon & apple spice sorbet 50
wholemeal flour 117
Wholemeal pecan pastry 108
Winter fruit salad 36

yoghurt, low-fat 115
Banana yoghurt pie 63–4
Blueberry yoghurt fruit swirls 55
Peach & yoghurt mousse 59